Angels In Italy

A True Story of a Cancer Survivor

S.D. HAYES

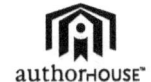

authorHOUSE™

1663 LIBERTY DRIVE, SUITE 200
BLOOMINGTON, INDIANA 47403
(800) 839-8640
WWW.AUTHORHOUSE.COM

First published by AuthorHouse 10/27/05

ISBN: 1-4208-8873-0 (sc)

Printed in the United States of America
Bloomington, Indiana

This book is printed on acid-free paper.

CHAPTER ONE

Life Is A Bowl Of Mixed Fruit

Susan would lie alone on the grass when she was a young girl and stare up at the clouds. She would imagine that someday a knight in shining armor would rescue her from her terrible stepfather's house and take her to his castle. Her real dad left when she was a baby and she didn't know him. When she was 3 years old her mom remarried and went to work everyday. She was the only stepchild in a family with four children. Bob, her cruel stepfather, and his family always made certain she knew she wasn't part of their family.

By the age of five she decided she didn't need them anyway. Her Uncle Dick loved her. She started flying all by herself from Oakland to Burbank, California. She loved to fly. The pretty flight attendants clipped a "Junior Stewardess" pin to her sweater. It was shaped into silver wings. Her pin made her feel so special she wore it every day.

Every summer vacation she spent with her mom's brother. It was a time before strict security at the airports and he could go out to the plane and meet her at the bottom of the stairs. He picked her up and twirled her around in a big hug. They went to Disneyland every year. During school she lived in the San Francisco Bay area but they moved a lot so Susan was never in one place long enough to make close friends.

She had no religious background except for the children's bible stories her mom read to her when she was very young. Occasionally she went to churches of different religions with schoolmates. She believed in God but deep down inside thought He was too busy to notice her.

As soon as she graduated from high school at age 17 she moved out to get away from her hateful stepfather. Her step-cousin and his wife were only a few years older than her and were always nice to her. They needed a babysitter so she moved in with them. In the evenings her cousin drove her to school so she could take classes. She saved every dime of her babysitting money for the next year and was thrilled to move into her very own apartment right after her 18th birthday.

She began her career in advertising with a newspaper in Oakland and her life changed. Her friends at the newspaper became her family. They grew up together, got married and had their babies together. She met her first husband Ron at the newspaper. He worked there also. He was 10 years older but she didn't care. He had blond hair, twinkling blue eyes and sent her flowers at work every single month.

When Susan turned 20 they got married in a little wedding chapel in Berkeley. They didn't have much money back then but neither did their friends. They made their home in Alameda and raised 2 sons. Her husband was the pitcher for a weekend baseball team. Susan took their young sons to all his games. Several members of a brand new football team in Oakland called the Raiders lived in Alameda and were on the baseball team.

Every Wednesday Susan met her mom and grandma for lunch at McDonalds. It was Grandma's treat. Her mom had worked at a bank in Oakland for as long as she could remember. It was only 2 blocks from the newspaper. The three of them had such fun being together. The sound of laughter from their table filled the lunchroom. Susan's mom was such a happy woman. She never understood why her mom stayed married to such a grouchy terrible man.

Susan always seemed to be in the right place at the right time when she worked for the newspaper. She met Governor Jerry Brown in the elevator at work. She asked him if he would come into her office to meet her friends and he did! He even put his arm around her like they were old friends.

John Voight was at the house across the street from theirs one Saturday campaigning for McGovern. When she saw him on the sidewalk as he walked out she invited him over for spaghetti. He politely thanked her but told her he had a plane to catch. Before he left he was nice enough to pose for a photo with her.

One afternoon she was walking down the stairs of the BART station. This was the new Bay Area Rapid Transit. As she was walking down she almost ran right into Prince Charles as he was walking up. They were face to face. What a shock! She shook his hand and said, "Welcome to Oakland." He was in northern California and wanted to ride on the new transportation. She hadn't even known he was in town.

While visiting an antique auction at the Fairmont Hotel in San Francisco with her girlfriend Sally she accidentally wandered into the ballroom and there was Robert Redford standing five feet in front of her! He was surrounded by a group of people. They were filming his new movie "The Candidate". Sally's headlights didn't work on her clunker car so the girls had to get back across the Bay Bridge before it got dark. Susan couldn't just walk away without saying something to him and couldn't think of a thing to say. She walked up to him, kissed him on the side of his mouth and boldly exclaimed, "Good-bye Darling, I have to leave now." He looked right into her eyes and quietly replied, "Come back when we can be alone." She almost melted into the parquet floor! Years later, when she happened to see him in a movie, she wondered what would have happened if she had come back.

Jane Fonda, Donald Sutherland and Peter Boyle were filming a movie around the corner from the newspaper. Susan happened to be walking by during her lunch hour and stopped to watch. The director came up to her and asked if she wanted to be in the movie. He said, "We need streetwalkers." She was surprised he asked her. She was 21 but still resembled Alice in Wonderland. She returned to work all excited with her news. Her boss let her go home early so she could make herself up to look like a hooker.

She returned later that evening wearing her suede mini skirt and high heels. Her hair was piled high and her eye makeup was thick. They had to wait until dark for the scene. Jane Fonda and Donald Sutherland invited Susan to join them in the bar where all the reporters hung out. She got to spend the next hour with them sitting around a small table talking. They were so nice to her and carried on just like ordinary people.

Susan's claim to fame was throwing a box of trash at Donald Sutherland as he ran down the street in Oakland chasing Jane Fonda. The movie, "Steelyard Blues" was fun and all her friends went to see it. About a month later Susan received a check in the mail from Steelyard Blues Productions for $12.00. It's a good thing she kept her daytime job!

Susan and Ron's marriage during the 70's was summer camping trips with kids and friends sitting around the campfire, frosty winter weekends in the mountains learning to ski, buying cheap furniture at flea markets, protesting the Viet Nam War and Oakland A's games at the Coliseum. Life was a bowl of cherries!

Suddenly, in the blink of an eye it was over. Susan's strong, healthy, young husband died of a heart attack when she was 28. The funeral was so huge their friends spilled out of the chapel and filled the street. The Alameda police had to close the road until the service was over. Susan was now a single mom.

She had to be strong and keep a happy face. She had two little sad sons who lost their dad. They needed every bit of her love. With no life insurance to help pay the bills, they moved to a more affordable small 2-bedroom house in Castro Valley where they lived for the next 17 years. It was important to Susan for her sons to stay in the same schools with the same friends until they finished high school.

It was difficult at times for the boys growing up without a dad but they had many happy years together in that little house. Susan continued working for the newspaper and had several second jobs to support her sons. She had learned that life is actually a bowl of mixed fruit. You get the sweet strawberries and cherries along with the sour grapes and lemons.

Susan had always dreamed of traveling and seeing more of the world. Her oldest son was grown now and living on his own. Her youngest son had just graduated from high school. They grew up to be fine young men. She knew from experience that we don't know how long we will have to enjoy life. We have to try to make all our dreams come true and never give up trying. It was time for her dream.

She retired from the newspaper after 15 years and totally changed careers. She started working in San Francisco for one of the largest U.S. airlines so she could fly free. The first trip she took with a friend was to England, France and Germany to visit real castles.

— CHAPTER TWO —

The Vision

Late one night in that twilight time between awake and asleep, Susan had a vision of an ancient splashing fountain with stone steps all around it. She felt happy and peaceful sitting on the steps in the sunshine watching two little girls with shining brunette hair. They were laughing as they chased each other around the fountain. Their white cotton dresses fluttered around little tan legs. Suddenly, Susan opened her eyes and sat upright in bed. She was instantly awake and alert. She felt she had just been in Rome, Italy. She had never even been to Rome before.

About a week later she had the same vision again while enjoying a lazy little nap on the couch on a Sunday afternoon. She opened her eyes and sat up against the pillows. Sunshine filled the cozy living room of her home but she felt she had just been outside in Rome. "How strange to have the same dream twice," she thought. "But it felt like much more than a dream. It actually felt like I was right there."

Monday morning she went back to work and soon forgot about the vision. She was working in international reservations. There was another price war going on between the airlines and she was too busy to think about anything but her job. She enjoyed working for the airline and had been there for several years.

The strangest thing happened the following week. She had the exact same vision a third time! It happened on a Saturday morning just as she was waking up in her bed. When she opened her eyes she could still feel the warmth of the sunshine on her face and the feel of cool stone on her palms from sitting on the steps of the fountain. Somehow she was positive this fountain was in Rome. She just knew it. She sat up and thought, "I have to go to Rome." She had a 2-week vacation coming up the next month.

The following weekend she visited a bookstore and bought a travel book about Italy. After reading the book she chose three cities to visit. First she would go to Florence, then Rome and finish her vacation in Venice. She started out feeling very excited but as the date grew near she started to chicken out. She thought to herself, "Are you crazy? You can't travel halfway around the world to a strange place by yourself!"

— CHAPTER THREE —

The Call

Then she received "the call" at work. It was just a routine call from a man confirming his flight from somewhere in Michigan with a connecting flight to Rome. He sounded like a friendly man so after confirming his flights and times she told him she was thinking about going to Rome soon for vacation also.

He asked her, "Have you been to Rome before?"

"No," she replied.

He asked, "Do you speak Italian?"

"No," she replied.

He then asked, "Do you have any hotel reservations?"

"No," she again replied.

After a brief pause he finally asked her, "Do you know anyone in Rome?"

Feeling a bit foolish now, she quietly replied, "No".

"Well, my dear," he said, "My name is Father Boyle. I

live in the Vatican and work in the Vatican library. Please write down my personal telephone number and call me if you have any trouble at all finding a place to stay. You are welcome to stay at the Vatican and I will give you a personal tour of the library."

She scribbled down his telephone number, thanked him for his kind offer, thanked him for choosing her airline, hung up the phone and then started shaking like a leaf!

All she could think was, "This must be a sign!" Her next immediate thought was, "I wonder if they make coffee in the mornings at the Vatican?" Crazy or not, she had to go to Rome. She could hardly wait for her lunch break so she could check the flights to Rome on her departure date. To fly free, employees had to go standby so the flights needed to have available seats.

Susan was so disappointed to find the flight to Rome was overbooked. She checked the following dates. They were full too. There was only 1 flight a day so she was out of luck. But then she thought, "After that call from Father Boyle I just have to get there!" She frantically began checking the flights on her computer to other big cities in Europe. Finally a breakthrough! She found available seats on a flight to Frankfurt, Germany. She would buy a Eurail pass and take the train from Frankfurt to Rome. She told herself, "No more thoughts of turning back now."

—◄ CHAPTER FOUR ►—

The Journey Begins

After the long flight to Frankfurt, Germany, Susan experienced a short moment of panic when she stood in the middle of the airport terminal surrounded by German speaking people and couldn't read a thing on any of the signs. Of course, they were written in German. She hadn't thought about that. Standing there like a lost child she thought, "I'm going to start crying in the middle of this airport. Think!" Then it came to her. Someone had once told her that if she ever felt lost in Europe to look for the big "I" sign for "Information". There it was, shining like a big blue beacon.

She walked over to the counter and asked the man behind the desk if he spoke English. He replied, "Of course! How may I help you?" With a sigh of relief and a happy smile Susan told him she needed to board a train to Florence, Italy. This kind man gave her the information she needed for the direct train to Florence. She wouldn't have to change trains. She thought, "Yes! I can do this alone!" She had already eaten on the plane so she didn't need German money for food. She could wait until she arrived in Italy to get Italian lira. As she walked over to her train platform she kept telling herself, "If I feel lonely or uncomfortable or lost, all I have to do is turn around and go back home."

With the "I" man's directions, she easily found the correct train and climbed aboard. After a short stroll down the aisle she found an empty compartment with two couches inside. Since this would be an overnight trip she thought a couch to stretch out on would be quite nice. It was a very nice compartment. The couches were comfortable with wide shelves above them where she could put her suitcase. The window was huge so she would have a perfect view of the country as the train whizzed by. There was a door to close for privacy when she slept later. This was going to be a great trip!

Susan had only been seated a few minutes and was looking out the window. She was feeling jet lagged from her long journey and was thinking about how nice it would be to sleep when the train started rolling. She jumped when she heard voices! She turned her head to see 3 Italian men entering her compartment. They looked a little startled when they saw her sitting there in the corner. They spoke to each other in Italian, shrugged then took the remaining seats on the couches. Susan had no idea this was a sleeping compartment that had to be reserved in advance. They hadn't entered her compartment… she was in theirs! As the train pulled away from the station, all Susan could think was, "Oh my God! I'm going to be spending the night on this train with 3 strange Italian men!"

As the train clattered along they all sat there in uncomfortable silence for about 30 minutes. Finally one of the men began a little shy conversation with her in Italian. She smiled and shook her head from side to side. With her hands spread she said, "I don't understand." When he heard her say this he spoke to her in timid English, "Where are you from?" She said, "I am an American traveling alone." He gave her a big smile and exclaimed, "Ah! You are American!" He paused for a moment then asked in an astounded voice, "You are traveling alone? Are you crazy?" She answered, "Yes! Yes!" They all looked amazed. Then they started laughing.

Now they all seemed quite excited to be able to practice their English with her. She learned two of them were uncle and nephew traveling home from a wedding. Their names were Ricardo and Edward. The other man was traveling home to his family from his job. His name was Frank. All the men took family photos from their wallets and proudly showed Susan their wives and children. When she told them this was her first time to Italy they excitedly began telling her all the places she should visit while in Florence, Rome and Venice.

To be of help to her, they all took out their lira and explained the amount of each coin. She showed them her American coins. This seemed to be quite a treat for them so she exchanged a few of her coins for theirs. They taught her how to say different phrases in Italian that she might need to know such as, "Avete una camera per una persona?" which means, "Do you have a room for one person?" As the train rattled across the German border into Italy, these caring men did everything they could think of to help her while she was in their country.

This new companionship they found with each other was beginning to feel quite comfortable for Susan until the hour grew late and everyone was becoming sleepy. She was thinking, "What's going to happen next?" Being familiar with this routine, the men stood and grabbed the suitcases off the shelves and stashed them under the couches. The upper shelves were then pulled out turning them into beds with mattresses. Their compartment was instantly transformed into a small bedroom with bunk beds on each side.

Susan just stood there, feeling quite awkward, trying not to get in their way. The men located bundles of sheets, blankets and pillows hidden in a closet in the aisle somewhere. Standing there with big smiles and arms full of linens they politely asked Susan, "Which bed would you prefer?" When they started taking off their shoes Susan decided this would be a good time to exit for the bathroom. She liked these guys but if they were going to take their pants off she didn't want to be around.

She lingered in the tiny bathroom at the end of the car long enough for them to get settled in bed. As she walked back down the aisle and approached the compartment she noticed they had closed the door. Feeling a little like an intruder, she quietly slid it open and tiptoed to her bed. She lay there stiff as a board and fully dressed with her blanket up to her chin. As she listened to her three companions breathing she thought for sure she would be awake all night. In about 2 minutes, with the soothing hypnotic sound of the train going click-clack over the tracks, she fell right to sleep.

As the brilliant sun rose over Italy, Susan awoke refreshed and hungry. She excused herself and took a walk to the bathroom to freshen up then began exploring the train to locate a restaurant car. It seemed odd to her but this train didn't have one. She stood in the aisle looking out the open window at the Italian countryside passing by and was awestruck by the beauty. The early morning sun was casting streaks of shadows between the trees onto the golden meadows.

She returned to her companions who had taken up the beds and were sitting on couches once again. The morning sun was shining through the window on their faces making them look as if they were glowing. They all smiled at her and exclaimed, "Buon Giorno!" which she had learned means, "Good Morning!"

They stood and opened their suitcases, pulling out paper sacks. They sat and lowered the tray which was hooked under the window. From their sacks they produced bread loaves, pastrami and cheese and made sandwiches on the tray. Obviously, they came prepared. When they handed Susan one of their sandwiches she thought she had never met such kind people.

Just then, a man pushing a trolley with snacks and coffee came down the aisle outside their compartment. The wonderful aroma of rich Italian coffee filled the air. She was dying for a morning cup of coffee! When her companions bought 4 cups and handed her one, she was thrilled and so grateful. As the foursome ate their sandwiches they chatted some more until the train arrived in Florence. When they began gathering their belongings from the overhead shelf Susan thanked them all for their kindness. They replied, "Ciao! Good luck crazy lady, Susanna!"

CHAPTER FIVE

Florence Italy

With no hotel reservations, Susan left the train station and began walking down a main street in Florence. The Italian name was Firenze. She wondered why Americans changed the name. As she practically skipped down Via De' Panzani, she pulled her suitcase behind her. Its wheels made a clicking sound rolling over the cobblestones. It was a glorious day. She had made it to Italy! She stopped at an ATM to get some lira then continued walking down the street in search of a hotel.

After only a few blocks she saw the La Gioconde Hotel sign. A round little Italian man was standing in front enjoying the sunshine. He smiled and greeted her with a friendly, "Buon Giorno!" She smiled and replied, "Buon Giorno! Do you speak English?" He said, "Yes, Are you looking for a hotel room?" She replied, "Yes". He told her he was the manager there. She asked him the price for a room. It was more than she wanted to spend. He then offered her his smallest single room with private bath. This was in her price range so she told him it would be perfect for her. With a hearty handshake, he introduced himself. His name was Fausto. Susan told him her name and said, "This is my first time visiting Florence." Fausto exclaimed, "Welcome!" Inside the lobby, he wrote down her passport information then gave her a map and circled all the places she should see.

Now that she had a place to stay and a city map of Florence, Susan was ready to start exploring this beautiful renaissance city. She spent the fresh spring morning wandering up and down the tiny streets on the north bank of the Arno River. She noticed the way the sun filtered down upon Florence somehow giving this city a pinkish glow and understood why artists have flocked to this remarkable city for centuries.

Florence was a great shopping town but very expensive. Susan stared into the swanky boutique windows at incredible leather jackets, skirts, shoes and handbags. Elegant designer dresses, silver pieces, gold jewelry and art prints tempted her everywhere.

Uffizi square was full of artists and souvenir stalls. She met an artist named Luigi when she paused to admire the picture he was painting. He spoke English. The day was becoming very warm and he invited her to sit in one of his folding chairs under his big shady royal blue umbrella. Luigi was gorgeous! Michelangelo would have wanted him to pose for a statue or paint his face in the Sistine Chapel. His face was that beautiful. Being such a hot day and all, of course Susan agreed to sit with him under his umbrella. He appeared to be in his late 30's, maybe 40. He was a young man so it seemed very odd and almost mystical when he began singing madrigal tunes quietly to himself as she watched him paint. Most guys she knew would be singing rock 'n roll or maybe an oldie but goodie song. Luigi was singing songs from the 16th, maybe 17th century. It was beautiful, almost hypnotizing.

She was fascinated watching him paint his picture of the square in Florence. After about 20 minutes of painting and quietly singing he put his brush down on the folding table next to him and asked her, "Will you join me for lunch?" Hmm, lunch with this gorgeous Italian? She supposed she could take a little more time from her sightseeing. Luigi pointed out different places of interest to Susan as they took a friendly walk around town. At an outdoor café they shared a late lunch. For the next 2 hours they sat at their small table talking. They asked questions about one another and their countries. They laughed and had a very nice time together. She offered to pay for her lunch but he insisted on buying.

As he walked her back to Uffizi square he told her he was playing his guitar that evening at a nearby club. He asked her if she could come to hear him play. For a brief moment she thought, "Should I stay in my room tonight or see Luigi again?" It wasn't too hard to decide! She told him she would come to the club. On the way back he pointed it out to her. After saying good-bye to Luigi she walked back to her hotel. It had been a long day of sightseeing and she wanted to rest before going out again that evening. Unfortunately, she fell asleep and didn't wake up until dawn. She felt bad for not going to the club when she told him she would but didn't have his phone number to call to apologize.

She got dressed and came downstairs. Fausto was sitting at the hotel desk. He looked up from his paperwork and gave her a beaming smile. They chatted about all the charming places she'd seen in Florence the day before. He asked her if she had ever seen the leaning tower of Pisa. She told him she hadn't. Fausto told her the train to the leaning tower of Pisa only took 1 hour. From the train station, the #1 bus would take her right to it. So off she went! She got there easily, just as he promised, and had lunch right next to the famous leaning tower.

When she returned, her friend Fausto gave her directions to walk to the Academy of Arts, which housed the famous statue of David by Michelangelo. It wasn't far, he said. What he forgot to tell her was that the streets changed names every block and she got quite lost. Like the crowded streets in downtown New York, the streets in Florence were teeming with people. Susan was completely confused and beginning to feel a bit panicky when, to her surprise and relief, Fausto seemed to appear right in front of her! She took his hands and exclaimed, "How did you find me?" He said, "When you didn't return I got worried and came looking for you."

Sweet Fausto took her to see David himself. After admiring David in all his perfect glory, they walked to the river Arno to see the ancient Ponte Vecchio Bridge built in the 1200's. He told her it was one of the few bridges to survive WWII. Little goldsmith shops, like a row of shoeboxes, lined the bridge. Their counters sparkled with delicate jewelry. Tourists crawled like ants all across the bridge.

They walked the short distance to the bus stop and hopped on a bus. He wanted her to see more of the sights in Florence. They drove by Palazzo Vecchio, a fortified palace. Fausto told her this was once the home of the Medici family who ruled Florence. After cruising past the extensive Boboli Gardens, the bus stopped at the beautiful Pitti Palace. They got off to go see it. It was closed that day so they wandered around the tree-shaded grounds. At the end of another long day, they took another bus to the top of the city. They climbed the stairs up to Piazzale Michelangelo Park for an incredible panoramic view of the glowing sunset and Florence with her golden domes. The city below them sparkled with twinkling lights.

The hotel had brochures in the lobby for day bus trips to various areas. That evening Fausto helped Susan make reservations for the following day to see 2 medieval towns. The bus picked her up at the hotel early the next morning. Most of her fellow passengers were from England, Germany and The Netherlands. Everyone spoke English.

First, they visited the beautiful walled city of San Gimignano. This wonderful Tuscan hill town still had 14 medieval towers from the original 72. It looked like a postcard setting. San Gimignano was built on top of a mountain in the 13th century. Feuding noble families would fight their battles from the protection of these tall towers. Years later, when fabric was their business, they would hang their yards of dyed fabric out to dry from the towers.

They drove on through the green and peaceful wine country to the ancient town of Siena. This medieval gem was built on 3 hills and divided into 17 neighborhoods called contradas. These small neighborhoods worshipped, competed and celebrated together. She learned about the famous Palio di Siena, a horse race held twice a year around the main square, Il Campo. Il Campo was in front of City Hall which had a 100-yard tall medieval tower. She learned that members from 10 of the chosen contradas race to be Numero Uno. Contrada pride was evident with different colorful banners fluttering from high windows giving Siena a very festive atmosphere. She hoped to return one day to see the Palio when Il Campo would be stuffed with locals and tourists.

After lunch at an outdoor café with classic European ambience, everyone toured the Duomo, Siena's cathedral. The busy interior was packed full with statues and ornamentation. The carved heads of 172 popes stared down at them from the ceiling. The group walked around Siena. Its traffic-free ancient narrow lanes curved every which way. As they wandered around, they peeked into charming courtyards with wells and climbing vines. They all had a great time on their tour.

They arrived back in Florence by early afternoon so Susan went for a walk and bought a gelato. She sat in the sunshine on the steps of the Duomo, the lovely cathedral covered with pink, green and white Tuscan marble, simply enjoying her ice cream and hanging out in Florence.

She finished her mocha flavored gelato cone before it could drip down her hand, then walked across to the Baptistery to see the famous bronze doors with 3-D like panels depicting bible scenes. These huge doors were incredible! The bronze glowed in the afternoon sunlight. She overheard a tour guide nearby saying a young man named Ghiberti finished the doors in 1452 after 24 years of labor. He was only 20 years old when he got this job. Michelangelo said these were fit to be the gates of Paradise.

On her last morning in Florence, Susan walked over to the Uffizi Gallery to see the great collection of Italian paintings inside. She bought a tour book on the street before entering. For the next 2 hours she wandered through the gallery on a self-guided tour. There weren't many tourists inside, mostly art students sketching. She admired 13th through 17th century masterpieces by great artists such as Rafael, Rubens, Botticelli and Michelangelo.

When she returned to check out of her hotel and say goodbye to her new friend Fausto, he asked where she was going next. She told him she was taking the train to Rome. "Do you have a hotel room reserved?" he asked. When she told him she didn't, he said he had a friend named Gian Luca who worked at the Hotel Igea in Rome. He asked, "Would you like me to call him and make a reservation for you?" She replied, "Yes! That would be great!" Fausto called Gian Luca. He had only one small room left and said he would save it for her. Susan thanked Fausto for all his help. He had taken such good care of her. She had never known a hotel manager to go out of his way to take care of a guest as Fausto did. She walked back to the train station. It was only a 2-hour ride to Rome.

Chapter Six

Rome

With Fausto's directions from the train station, Susan found the Hotel Igea easily. The woman at the desk told her Gian Luca wasn't there but he had saved the last room for her. The maids were still cleaning it so Susan left her suitcase with the woman and went for a walk to a nearby café for a cappuccino.

As she sat at the small table in the afternoon sunshine studying the map of Rome she had purchased at the train station, the man sitting at the next table said something to her in Italian. She said, "I'm sorry, I don't understand." He exclaimed, "You are from California!" When she asked him how he knew, he said, "I could tell by your accent." He couldn't help but notice her map spread on the table and asked if he could help. She told him she had just arrived. He happily talked about the places she must see while in Roma and circled them on her map. He then introduced himself.

His name was Lorenzo. She told him her name. He looked like a businessman and was very friendly and polite. He told her he owned a small restaurant around the corner and invited her to be his guest for dinner that evening. She certainly didn't have any plans for dinner so she agreed to go.

When she arrived later that night, Lorenzo met her at the door and showed her to a table. He looked very happy to see her. He said, "I am preparing my special pasta dish for you!" All during dinner he treated her like she was a celebrity. He didn't want her to feel alone or uncomfortable so every few minutes he would come to her table to see if she was happy and enjoying her pasta.

There was a nicely dressed elderly gentleman eating his dinner at the next table. When he finished, he asked Lorenzo something in Italian. Lorenzo returned with a banana on a china plate. She watched, out of the corner of her eye, as the gentleman peeled his banana very carefully with his knife. He then proceeded to carefully cut the banana into small pieces with his knife and fork and eat it very slowly with his fork. For some reason, this cracked her up! She had never seen anyone make such a big production out of eating a banana before. This kept her secretly entertained for quite some time.

After her wonderful dinner, she thanked Lorenzo and asked him for the check. He insisted there was no charge. He said, "You are my special guest!" He then asked her if she would join him for dancing. He had been very gracious to her all evening so she agreed to go. She was glad she had brought her turquoise suede skirt and jacket on the trip so she had something nice to wear.

Lorenzo drove her to a small elegant club nearby. A valet parked the car. They entered and were shown to a table for two by the dance floor. After ordering 2 glasses of wine, Lorenzo asked her to dance. A man in a tuxedo was playing a grand piano. The music sounded like a beautiful Italian love song. After the dance they returned to their table. They had a good time talking together. Lorenzo then excused himself and walked over to say something to the piano player. Suddenly, to her delight, he played "I left my heart in San Francisco" for her. After an enjoyable evening, Lorenzo drove her back to her hotel. In the car, he gave her his business card and told her to call him if she needed any help. He said, "I hope you have a wonderful holiday in Roma." She thanked him for his kind offer and for a wonderful evening. On the way back, he drove by the Vatican and the Colosseum so she could see them for the first time aglow at night. What an unbelievable sight!

Back in the lobby of her Hotel Igea, she met Fausto's friend Gian Luca for the first time. He was behind the hotel desk. He was a cute Italian and looked about 30. His hair and eyes were very dark brown and he had a sweet smile. He said, "I'm very happy to meet you. How is your room?" She told him it was very nice and thanked him for saving the last one for her. He said, "If you need any help while you are in Roma, please let me know. I will be happy to help you." She excitedly rattled on to him about her sightseeing plans for the next day. He told her when she visited Trevi Fountain to be sure to throw in coins. With a twinkle in his eye, he said, "Throw one coin and you will return to Roma, two coins and you will fall in love with someone in Roma."

Early the next morning Susan left her hotel with her map, excited to begin exploring. Most of the places Lorenzo had circled on her map were within walking distance in the old core of Roma. On her way to Trevi Fountain, she saw people sitting at outdoor cafes. They were smiling and talking to one another excitedly with their hands waving around. Between the small shops, hotels and restaurants were ancient Roman ruins with excavations still going on. They just built the new around the old and created a kind of chaotic harmony. It was love at first sight for Susan!

She wandered past beautifully displayed colorful fresh fruit and vegetable stands. Round women with baskets hung over their arms were choosing perfect pieces for their meals. There were carved stone splashing fountains and small piazzas at every turn. Young couples were kissing. Chic women rode bicycles. Small bakeries had wonderful pastries displayed in front windows. The aroma of freshly baked bread floated out their doorways. The crazy traffic jammed the streets and cars were honking. Motor scooters buzzed around the cars, like flies. It was crazy, exciting and beautiful all at the same time! She smiled and thought, "To be walking down the streets of this ancient, incredible city is like a beautiful dream!" She felt in her heart like she had come home, as if she belonged right here.

When she arrived at the sparkling Trevi Fountain she remembered what Gian Luca had told her. She smiled and threw 2 coins in over her shoulder. She sat on the steps in front of the fountain in the Roman sunshine for quite awhile just soaking it all up, the beauty, the history and the remarkable feeling she had to be alive at this place, at this time.

CHAPTER SEVEN

The Day That Changed Susan's Life

From Trevi Fountain, she walked to the Piazza di Spagna, known as the Spanish Steps because it was once the site of the Spanish Embassy. College students with backpacks were sitting on the steps. Some of them were studying but most were simply talking to one another and enjoying the sunshine. Susan walked past them up the steps to the very top. She stopped to admire some watercolor landscape paintings for sale. They were displayed on easels. She told the man selling the paintings, "They are beautiful." He said, "Thank you. Are you American?" She replied, "Yes, I am from California."

With a brilliant smile he introduced himself. He said, "My name is Giovanni Giovanetti. What is your name?" She smiled back. His name had rolled off his tongue in seven syllables. She said, "My name is Susan. This is my first day in Roma." With great enthusiasm he exclaimed, "I have lived in Roma all of my life and I want to show you all of my favorite places!" This was the day that changed Susan's life. It was May 28, 1992.

Giovanni put the paintings in his car and made a call from his cell phone. He took the rest of the day off to be with her. The excitement and glowing pride he had for his home spread to Susan in a way she had never felt from anyone before. He took her hand in his and they spent the day loving his beautiful city.

They walked to Campo dei Fiori, a bustling outdoor flower and produce market. The delicious aromas of fresh herbs and flowers filled the market square. They picked out juicy fresh fruit to eat while they walked. They wandered through Piazza Navona, a lively square with three ornately carved fountains by Bernini. He showed her the "Sacred Area", an excavation pit with some of the oldest ruins in Rome. He told her Julius Caesar was assassinated here.

They visited the ancient Pantheon. Giovanni told her it became a church dedicated to the martyrs after the fall of Rome. The dome was 140 feet high with a hole in the center. He said because of this, many Romans believe it was built as an ancient observatory. As they stood under the portico outside, he told her the gigantic one-piece granite columns were shipped from Egypt.

In Michelangelo's Renaissance Square they admired his beautifully designed staircase. As Giovanni shared his Roma with Susan they always held hands and walked side by side. He had a jaunty step when he walked and a contagious joy for life. He shared his knowledge with her about all the history she was seeing for the first time.

Leisurely, they wandered through the ancient Forum then went inside the Colosseum to sit on the steps to rest. Here on these 2000 year old steps they sat a long while and talked non-stop, wanting to learn everything there was to know about one another. She learned that he wasn't the artist who painted the watercolor landscapes, as she had previously thought. His roommate and best friend was the artist. He was only there that day because his friend had an appointment and asked him to help out in the morning. Giovanni worked in the Vatican offices. His dream was to one day be a fashion designer.

She asked him how he learned to speak English so well. He told her he learned from the tourists and from watching American movies. His knowledge of the English language wasn't always perfect though. When she asked him if he was a good cook he replied, "I used to be but my ex-wife took my chicken." When she finally controlled her laughter she told him the correct word was kitchen.

— CHAPTER EIGHT —

The Fountain

That evening Giovanni told her he was taking her to his favorite area of Roma called Piazza Santa Maria in Trastevere. Susan had never heard of this area. They walked across a bridge and along several narrow streets. They passed open windows with families inside. They could hear happy sounding Italian conversations and smell the fresh basil from Mama's cooking floating out of their windows. Freshly washed laundry fluttered on the clotheslines, which were strung between the buildings above their heads. They continued on into this very old and charming part of the city.

When they arrived at the Piazza, Susan suddenly stopped and stared. There, in the center of Piazza Santa Maria in Trastevere, was the exact fountain she had the visions of before she had ever been to Italy! Tears glistened in her eyes. She felt like the world had suddenly stopped. Giovanni just put his arms around her and held her. They stood there in the Piazza holding each other for a long time, not even noticing the other people that swirled by around them.

Giovanni didn't ask her why she suddenly felt so emotional. Somehow he knew this was where she was supposed to be. He took her hand and led her inside the ancient church named Santa Maria in Trastevere. Sitting inside together in the hushed dim lighting he quietly told her this was one of Roma's oldest churches. It was made a basilica in the 4th century when Christianity was legalized. He said most of what she was seeing was from the 12th century. Susan was so enchanted by this lovely little church and the man who introduced it to her.

When they emerged from the church, the sunset had turned the skies above Roma into a bright shade of tangerine with pink swirls. The restaurants surrounding the small piazza had turned on their twinkling white lights. Susan and Giovanni found an outdoor table for two and ordered spaghetti and red wine. The savory aromas of garlic, herbs and rich sauces floated around them on this warm spring evening.

She finally told him about her vision of this fountain. She thought he might think she was crazy but he didn't at all. As they sat there across from each other at the small table he held both of her hands in his and looked deep into her eyes. He watched her smile as if he were memorizing her every emotion. She looked back at Giovanni's face. He wasn't gorgeous but he had a nice face. He had a proud Roman nose, beautiful full lips and eyes that seemed to see into her very soul. They talked the entire evening getting to know one another more. As the sky became a deep purple and the stars began to twinkle above them, an accordion player nearby began to play and sing a lovely Italian love song.

A darling round older man with a big mustache and a basket full of long-stem red roses walked up to their table. Giovanni bought one, stood up and gallantly handed it to Susan. A single red rose makes a woman feel so special. She smiled and gave him a tiny kiss on his lips. His beautiful smile lit up his face.

After their long leisurely dinner he walked her back to her hotel. He had to get up early for work the next day. He asked her what her plans were for the next day. She told him she wanted to visit the Vatican. He said he wished he could be her tour guide but he had to work. She felt such happiness when he said, "I want to see you again." She told him she wanted to see him again too. They agreed to meet the next day at 3:00 at the Spanish Steps.

CHAPTER NINE

Have You Ever Seen A Light Walking?

Bright and early the next morning Susan came down-stairs and asked Gian Luca how to get to the Vatican. He was very helpful and told her to take the #64 bus and where to catch it. Before she left she called Father Boyle but was disappointed to learn he wasn't working that day or the next. This was her only regret while in Italy. She wanted to meet him and thank him personally for his kind offer to help her. Unfortunately, they had not discussed specific dates. Susan took the bus with no problems to the Vatican.

St. Peter's Basilica was the most impressive church on earth. She felt like a dwarf standing inside with her head craned heavenward. The vastness and richness of St. Peter's was truly beyond anything she could have imagined. She spent over an hour inside walking around to see everything. It was definitely awesome but didn't quite feel like a super holy place to her because there were hundreds of tourists talking loudly and taking flash pictures. She thought how lovely it would feel to be alone inside. Another 4 hours were spent shuffling through the Vatican Museum and beautiful Sistine Chapel. When she finished her tour, she took the bus to her hotel and walked back to the Spanish Steps to meet Giovanni.

She instantly spotted him in the crowd the same moment he saw her. With a huge smile on his face, he rushed over to her. He gave her a big hug and exclaimed, "I was afraid you had just been a dream!" He asked her if she wanted to take a drive to the beach. This sounded like fun so she said, "Yes." They quickly walked over to his nearby small economy car and took off. He was a crazy Italian driver, honking just like all the others. Before they left the city, Giovanni drove her by the Circus Maximus to show her the sight of the ancient chariot races. It amazed her that it was still there.

It took them about an hour to drive to the beach. The time went by quickly because they talked to each other the entire trip. They found a parking place and took off their shoes in the car. For the next 3 hours they held hands and talked as they made footprints in the sand beside the incoming frothy waves. She told him she had 2 grown sons at home named Rick and Erin. He said he also had a son, a 6-year old named Simone. He asked her if she would like to meet him. She told him she would love to. He said he would make arrangements with his ex-wife to pick him up the next day.

That evening they walked back to Piazza Santa Maria

in Trastevere for another beautiful dinner outside under the luminous stars. The man selling roses was there again and Giovanni bought Susan another long-stem red rose. The restaurants in the piazza filled with smiling Italian families talking to each other with great enthusiasm. With Giovanni, Susan felt like she was a part of this big happy family called Roma.

As they were walking back to Susan's hotel that night, Giovanni suddenly asked, "Have you ever seen a light walking?" She had no clue what he was talking about and thought he must be using an incorrect English word. He let go of her hand and ran ahead, bent down and scooped something up. Walking back to her, he had a grin on his face and his hands were cupped together like he was praying. She wondered, "What is this silly man up to?" He had her hold both her hands up to his and take his surprise into her own hands. To her utter amazement, she peeked inside and there was a firefly glowing in her hands. She had never in her life seen one before. It felt like magic!

— CHAPTER TEN —

Meeting A Little Cherub

The next morning Giovanni picked Susan up at her hotel and little Simone was in the backseat. What a doll! He had the sweet face of a little cherub. They drove to Tivoli Gardens. Giovanni told Susan the story about the gardens. He said, "A man, so much in love with his new bride, had a house built for her here. She loved fountains so he filled the gardens surrounding their home with all different types of ornate fountains to make her happy." That was long ago and the area was open to the public now.

The three of them walked all around the lush gardens and sat by the splashing fountains as Susan and Simone became acquainted. Giovanni told her that children are taught English in Italian schools beginning at age seven. Simone was only six. He understood English pretty well from his father but was still quite shy about speaking it. It was amazing how well they could communicate though with smiles and hand gestures. Giovanni helped Susan with Italian words and helped Simone with English words.

From Tivoli Gardens, they drove to a small outdoor restaurant for lunch where Susan had her first salmon pizza. It was wonderful. Covering the thin crust was thinly sliced salmon smothered with some type of hot bubbly white cheese. After lunch, they drove to Villa Borghese, Rome's "Central Park". Simone's bicycle was stashed in the trunk of the car. The park had nice paved pathways for him to ride his bike. While Susan and Giovanni lay on their backs on the green grass under the sprawling oak trees, Simone got to show them all of his bike tricks. What a day they shared full of laughter.

At the end of the afternoon, Giovanni's ex-wife met them at the park to pick up little Simone. Susan was a bit nervous about this meeting but Giovanni's ex-wife seemed genuinely interested in meeting this American woman who was making Giovanni so happy. She was very warm and friendly and the meeting was comfortable. Giovanni told Susan later that he and his ex-wife had decided they didn't want to be married to each other anymore but agreed to stay friendly for their son. She had a boyfriend and was happy. She wanted him to be happy too.

CHAPTER ELEVEN

Was It The Magic Of Roma?

They went back to Piazza Santa Maria in Trastevere for dinner that evening, but this time instead of heading to a table, Giovanni led Susan to the fountain. They sat on the ancient steps holding hands. It was a quiet time to embrace the mood. They listened to the buzz of people around them and watched the water droplets from the fountain as they sparkled like crystals in the late afternoon sunshine. Their time together was coming to an end. Susan was taking the train to Venice the next day to spend the last five days of her Italy vacation.

Slowly, Giovanni turned to look into Susan's eyes. He took both of her hands in his and said, "I don't want to lose you. I love you. Will you marry me?" Susan looked back into his eyes. She smiled and quietly said, "Yes."

It was that simple. Right there, at the fountain of her dreams in the heart of Rome, they both knew it was right.

Susan had been single for 15 years and had only known this man for a few days but she didn't even have to think it over before she said yes. Was it the magic of Roma? She felt as if she had finally come home and Giovanni was the other half of her that she'd been searching for her whole life. He felt exactly the same about her.

Was there electricity in the air in Piazza Santa Maria in Trastevere that evening? Or were the sparkles coming from the two of them? As they sat there at their small table talking with so much enthusiasm about their future, the man with the roses came by their table again. Giovanni bought Susan another red rose. He excitedly babbled to the rose man in Italian. He told him, "I have just asked this woman to marry me and she said yes!" Their waiter overheard this and told the other waiter. Soon everyone around them in the little outdoor restaurant was smiling at them and babbling in Italian!

Susan asked Giovanni if he could come with her to Venice. He said he wanted to but had to ask if he could get some holiday time off from work. He told her when he was a boy his family always took vacations to Venice and he hadn't been back in years. They decided to meet the next day at noon after he talked to his supervisor about the time off.

After dinner on that warm lovely evening they walked hand in hand all around Rome. The ancient ruins, statues and fountains were aglow from amber spotlights. At the Spanish Steps, people were sitting and enjoying the warm evening. Susan and Giovanni walked up the steps and sat down amidst them. There were mostly college students but also a nice mixture of older married couples, even some tourists from other parts of the world.

One of the students began playing old Beatles songs on his guitar. When he played "Hey Jude", a few of the students began singing and everyone joined in. His next song was John Lennon's, "Imagine". As they all sang the sweet lyrics to this, Susan thought about how perfect it all was. Here they were, from all walks of life, from different countries, singing the beautiful words of "Imagine" in harmony. It was one of those special moments in her life that she would carry in her heart forever.

As Giovanni walked Susan back to her hotel, he told her he had some holiday time off in September and wanted to come to California to be with her and see where she lived. She said she wanted to return to Rome soon to be with him again too. They hadn't had time yet to make any definite plans. They just knew they had to be together. They had faith they would somehow make it work.

Susan spent the next morning meandering around Rome. It was her last day and she wanted to absorb every detail of this city she had quickly grown to love. She walked over to the Spanish Steps at noon to meet Giovanni. The minute he saw her he started running. He had a happy smile on his face. When he caught up to her, he grabbed her and spun her around. He exclaimed, "I have the rest of today and the next 4 days off. We're going to Venice together!" He had already packed his bag and was ready to go.

As excited as two kids off to summer camp, they drove to Susan's hotel to get her things. Gian Luca was very protective and wouldn't let Giovanni go up to the room with her. This seemed very unusual to Susan. Gian Luca was too young for this old world way of thinking but he insisted on protecting her. She was surprised but also felt cherished. She went upstairs alone and quickly packed her bag. When she rejoined Giovanni downstairs, she thanked her friend Gian Luca for all his help and said goodbye. With her roses in hand and their bags in the backseat, they drove to the train station. Giovanni had already checked the departure time for the train to Venice and reserved a hotel. He bought his ticket and they boarded the train.

CHAPTER TWELVE

The Wonder Of Venice

The train ride might have taken two hours or perhaps four? They were so involved with each other, talking and laughing, Susan didn't notice the time. When they arrived at the Venice train station, they located a water taxi called a vaporetto. Off they went, skimming through the water, to the area of Venice where their hotel was reserved. Hotel Alloggi Alle Scale was in a very quiet location at the end of a narrow lane. Their room was decorated with antique furniture, accented by a cheerful white fabric with red poppies. Right next-door was a perfect little gold and white petite palace with a spiral staircase winding up the front.

As soon as they dropped their bags in the room they set out hand in hand for a lazy sunset passaggiata walk to enjoy the end of the warm afternoon. Susan and Giovanni could hardly wait to begin exploring ancient Venice together for the first time.

The very first thing Susan noticed was the still sweet quietness. With no noisy cars buzzing around, she could hear the birds all around her having a conversation. With no car exhaust fumes the air was springtime fresh. It was like a journey back in time to unhurried days and innocent times. She saw other couples enjoying their leisurely stroll. Window boxes were spilling over with green vines and bright red geraniums on brightly painted old dwellings with Byzantine architecture. Little tables at outdoor cafes were full of smiling people relaxing and taking time to enjoy talking with one another.

The many, many canals, oh the canals! Shiny black lacquer gondolas glided quietly by. The men controlling the boats were dressed in tight black pants with black and white striped shirts. Using a long pole to push them quietly along, some of them sang as they drifted by. Their beautiful voices were echoing under the small arched bridges. The water sparkled in the sunshine as if tiny diamond chips were floating along.

As the sun was setting, they walked along narrow winding streets until they found a charming little outdoor restaurant. Small tables with red and white-checkered tablecloths were set up under a bright red awning. Surrounding the tables were leafy green potted plants. The sweet sound of accordion music, played by a man strolling near the tables, set the mood. They enjoyed a delicious meal with candlelight and a bottle of red wine.

They began with bruschetta, toast brushed with olive oil, garlic and tomatoes. They both ordered Tortellini ai funghi, a small c-shaped pasta filled with meat and smothered with porcini mushrooms, butter, cream and fresh parmesan. Susan was surprised when, at the end of their meal, their waiter asked her if she would like salad. Giovanni explained that in Italy, they ate their salad at the end of the meal. Susan thought this made sense, really, so the meal wouldn't get cold. For dessert, they shared a profiterole, a cream-filled pastry with chocolate sauce.

Here in Venice, another man walked up to their table selling roses. Giovanni bought another red rose for "My Susanna", an endearing name he had begun to call her. After a wonderful dinner, they walked over to the main square in Venice, the incomparable Piazza San Marco.

The architecture of the buildings on one side of the Piazza was Renaissance from the 16th century. On the opposite side was 17th century Baroque. These majestic buildings were aglow at night with small white lights strung up along the rooflines. Pricey shops and small cafes were tucked under arches along the first floors. Golden domes and pointed spires crowned the church of San Marco. The tower of Campanile di San Marco stood 300 feet tall. The lagoon at the end of Piazza San Marco was lined with gondolas tied to wooden poles which were painted in bright blue and white stripes.

The exquisite beauty of Piazza San Marco thrilled Susanna. It was nearly 2 football fields long. They walked the length of it to the end where 2 outdoor orchestra stages were set up. They were adorned with pale pink long billowing draperies. The orchestra members looked very elegant in their tuxedos as they prepared their instruments. All the pigeons left to go sleep wherever it is that pigeons go to sleep at night. One of the orchestras began to play. Giovanni asked Susanna to dance. Right there under the stars, in the middle of Piazza San Marco, Europe's most romantic dance floor, just the two of them danced and danced. They twirled around the piazza like two figures on a music box.

— CHAPTER THIRTEEN —

Discovery

At the end of a perfect evening they walked back along the dimly lit narrow streets to their small hotel, each so happy with their newly found love. Inside their room, locked away from the rest of the world, they kissed. Sweet gentle loving kisses quickly became very intense, as if their spirits were joining. Their hands slowly began to discover each other's bodies.

The very instant Giovanni gently put his hand under Susanna's blouse to her breast he abruptly stopped and backed away from her. He looked right into her surprised eyes and said, "What's wrong with you?"

Her first thought was, "He's got his words in the English language screwed up." She asked him, "What do you mean, what's wrong with me?" His eyes had an alarmed look in them when he said, "You have a small ball of grass." Now he really lost her. She had no idea what he was talking about.

He became very frustrated with himself because he didn't know the correct English word for what he was trying to tell her. He tried again but his stream of words was in Italian. She just stood there looking at him. With a concerned look on his face, he slowed down his words and said, "My ex-mother-in-law had a small ball of grass in her breast and she died."

The poor man looked so upset. Susanna hugged him and assured him nothing was wrong with her. She told him, "My mother died from cancer many years ago. Because of this, I go to the doctor every year for a pap smear and the doctor always gives me a breast exam. I also have a mammogram every single year." She wasn't quite sure if he understood all of this. After all, words like "mammogram" aren't English words you use in everyday conversations. After all her confident words of reassurance, he still made her promise to go to the doctor as soon as she returned home. She promised him she would.

Talk about ruining the moment! Fortunately, the dreamy kissing and hugging began again and they quickly forgot all about this conversation. For the next 4 sizzling nights they made passionate love. When he whispered to her in Italian while they were in bed, it absolutely gave her goose bumps. They quietly talked to each other afterwards about their feelings and dreams, long into the wee hours. The love and desire they felt for one another became brighter, more intense, more dazzling with each moment they spent together.

One of the other pleasures of Venice for both of them

was walking its serpentine passageways, each revealing its own surprises. With 100 islands connected by 400 sweet bridges, Venice was a wonderland to them. Every day was a new adventure as they roamed all over Venice exploring this grand ancient city of palaces, canals and wonderful food. They must have been absolutely glowing. Everywhere they went, people would look at them and smile.

— CHAPTER FOURTEEN —

Delightful Moments In Venice

With the wind in their hair and grins on their faces, they stood at the railing on a ferry headed for Murano Island. On this small island, they watched with fascination as sweaty men demonstrated their glass blowing talents before red-hot furnaces. This skill was passed down to them from their fathers and grandfathers. Murano is a pretty little island with trees and shady lanes to wander along. Brightly colored exquisite Murano glass pieces glittered in the windows of the many tiny shops built in a row along the canals.

Carciofi Panini was on the menu in front of a small café. Susanna asked Giovanni what it was. After thinking for a moment of the word in English, he said, "Artichoke sandwiches." They bought two and walked over to the nearby church. Sitting on the church steps in the sunshine, they enjoyed their tasty lunch. The artichoke sandwiches were delicious. They laughed as they watched the flirty male white pigeons fluff up and dance around the females.

They also visited the lovely island of Burano. As they strolled around this sleepy little island, they stopped many times to watch old women making delicate lace. Giovanni bought Susanna another red rose from a lovely little flower stand at the water's edge.

Every single day, since the first day they met, Giovanni bought his Susanna a long-stem red rose. Each one was in a tiny vile of water so, amazingly, they were all still fresh and beautiful. He made her feel like she was the most special woman in the whole world. She adored him.

One afternoon Giovanni stopped in front of a small gift shop and wanted to go inside. Susanna wasn't about to argue with a chance for shopping. While she was buying souvenirs for friends at home, he went to another area of the shop. He secretly bought her a ring with a small crystal blue stone, the color of the sky in Venice. They left the shop with their gift bags dangling from their arms and walked over to Piazza San Marco for cappuccinos.

Seated at a small café table under a big green umbrella, Susanna cried when Giovanni took her hand and slipped the ring onto her finger. He gently wiped the tears from her cheeks and said, "I will buy you a better ring later but for now, I want you to wear this ring to remind you of how much I love you." She would always cherish that little ring.

The following day they hopped on another ferry to San Lazzard, a lovely monastery island. After visiting the old monastery, they sat on a bench at the water's edge. In the cool dappled shade of a huge tree, probably as ancient as the monastery itself, they gazed out at the water and distant islands. It was so quiet and peaceful here. It actually felt like a special mystical place. For hours they quietly talked about how remarkable it was that they had found one another and about their wonderful future together.

Later that evening, back in the city, they got quite lost in the tangle of tiny streets. The sliver of sky above them, between the buildings, was pitch black. The dim lighting coming from the small restaurants scattered here and there didn't help much. All the streets they walked down began to look alike in the dark. Addresses were hopelessly confusing. After wandering around in circles a few times they finally started laughing. They were on an island, how lost could they be? Giovanni finally stopped someone and asked for directions to their street. Even Italian men in Italy are forced to ask directions occasionally.

For their last dinner in Venice they found their way to the Grand Canal. At an outdoor restaurant by the famous Rialto Bridge, built in 1592, they were seated at a table right next to the water. They had a perfect view of the gondolas gliding by in the canal. As the late afternoon sun began to set and Venice was filled with a warm golden shimmering glow, 4 gondolas pulled up side-by-side in front of them. All 4 men began to sing a beautiful Italian love song. Their voices echoed off the ancient buildings sounding as clear as a concert stage. It was perfect.

A hot loaf of fresh bread was brought to their table while

they were waiting for their dinner. There were small sparrows perched on one of the shiny gondolas tied up to a red and white striped pole in the water below. Susanna took a tiny piece of crust and put it in her open palm. A brave little sparrow flew over and landed on her palm. He lingered there quite relaxed, pecking at the piece of bread. Giovanni smiled. It was just another delightful moment in Venice.

This was their last night together in Venice. With a quiet sadness, holding hands across the table, they gazed at one another memorizing every detail of each other's faces. Giovanni's eyes looked so sad and serious. They trusted they would be together again. Giovanni bought his Susanna another red rose. He handed it to her and said, "I will love you forever."

— CHAPTER FIFTEEN —

The End Of A Perfect Vacation

They stayed awake most of that night in their big fluffy bed cuddling, touching, loving, talking, smiling, kissing, neither one of them wanting the morning light to end their time together. As they sat in bed, Susanna asked Giovanni to design some dresses for her. He grabbed some paper and a pencil and sketched 5 different designs in about 5 minutes. He was really quite talented. Sometime in the wee hours of the morning, they finally fell asleep in each other's arms. All too soon, the new day arrived. They wanted so much to cover their heads with the blanket and ignore the morning sun but they had trains to catch.

A short vaporetto ride took them back to the train station. Susanna's train to Frankfurt left an hour before Giovanni's train to Rome. On the train platform, they stood holding each other as long as they could. After promising to be together again soon, Susanna climbed the train steps with her suitcase and her huge bouquet of red roses. Her heart was breaking. She felt like she was leaving half of herself behind in Italy. She found a seat by an open window. Giovanni stood outside holding her hand. They both had tears streaming down their faces as they let go and the train pulled away.

The customs official at the Frankfurt airport had no romance in his heart. He wouldn't let Susanna take her roses. She knew she would always keep them bundled up in her heart though. On the long flight home she thought of Giovanni and cried and smiled. She felt so sad and so very happy at the same time. She was still amazed that she had traveled all the way to Italy and found the one man, out of all the people in Rome, she wanted to spend the rest of her life with. Giovanni knew they belonged together and so did she.

She closed her eyes on the plane and remembered Italy and the kind people she had met. She would treasure these memories forever. No one had ever tried to take advantage of a woman traveling alone. She had come alone but was never alone. Everyone she met had been so warm and friendly, protective towards her and always helpful.

— CHAPTER SIXTEEN —

Susanna Reunited With Giovanni!

Susanna returned to San Francisco in June and went back to work. Giovanni called her every single night and told her how much he missed her. He reminded her to make a doctor appointment. She really hadn't given it another thought. He wouldn't let it go so she made an appointment for the following month towards the end of July.

At work, she was busily trading days off with co-workers so she could return to her Giovanni. Everyone was more than willing. She told them she had fallen in love with a Roman and they were all excited for her. She worked through her days off so she could return to Rome for a week. Giovanni also worked things out to get the time off work. Over the phone he exclaimed, "I told my family all about you. I told them we are getting married. They are happy for us and are looking forward to meeting you."

The day finally arrived when Susanna could return to

Giovanni. This time she was able to get on a stand-by flight direct from San Francisco to Rome. However, because she was so excited to get there, the flight seemed to take forever. When the plane finally landed, it took an eternity to get through customs. Giovanni was waiting for her just on the other side of the wall and she couldn't see him yet. When she finally got to walk through that doorway and turn the corner, the laughter just bubbled out of her. There was her Giovanni jumping up and down behind the crowd of people with a huge smile and a bouquet of 17 long-stem perfect red roses! He bought one for every day they had been apart. The crowd of people parted and she ran into his open arms. They stood right there in the middle of the Leonardo da Vinci Airport kissing and hugging.

Giovanni had reserved a lovely room for them near the Spanish Steps. Needless to say, they could hardly wait to get to their room and be alone together. The passion and electricity between them was so intense. The gentleness, touching and quietly talking long into the night afterwards was pure love.

Rome in July was very hot and humid. They spent leisurely summer days at the beaches of Delfino and Fiumicino. They drove to Castel Gondolfo Lake, where the Pope has a summer home, to enjoy the cooler countryside. A couple of steamy afternoons were spent together in Villa Borghese Park in Rome, just lying on the cool grass under big shady green trees that were gnarled with age like fairy tale gnomes. They talked and talked, wanting to know more and more about each other. Always holding hands and touching, Giovanni and Susanna just couldn't get enough of each other.

When they walked to cafes, they would always stop at the many beautiful stone fountains scattered throughout Rome. As was the local custom in the July heat, they would sit on the edge of the fountain squished between all the other Italians. With their feet in the cool sparkling water they would slowly kick their legs like two happy kids on a summer afternoon.

They took little Simone with them to the park one afternoon so he could ride his bike. At the time, Ninja Turtles were all the rage with the kids in the U.S. Susanna bought some to take to Simone. Little Simone knew what Ninja Turtles were. In fact, he knew all their names. He was very excited with her gifts. He hugged her and rattled on to her a-mile-a-minute about each of them. She couldn't understand what he was saying in Italian, all she could see was how happy he was. His initial shyness was gone and they became very comfortable with each other. When Simone put his little hand in hers as they walked through the park she felt so loved and accepted. He was the sweetest little thing. How could she not love him?

— CHAPTER SEVENTEEN —

Meeting The Family

It was time to meet the rest of the family. Giovanni's mother wanted to cook a big dinner for Susanna to welcome her into the family but the weather was way too hot to be in the kitchen. Instead they decided to meet for dinner at an outdoor restaurant. Susanna was a little nervous about the meeting, hoping they would accept a foreigner into their family. She needn't have worried. They met her with open arms! Giovanni's parents, Adili and Frederico, insisted immediately that she call them Mama and Papa. Giovanni's brother, Maurizio and his lovely wife, Patricia, were also there with their teenage son, Fabrizio. With beaming smiles, they all hugged her and gave her a kiss on each cheek. She almost cried she was so happy! Never had she been made to feel so welcome.

And never had she been served so much food! They all sat outside at a long table. When Papa opened the wine,

Patricia handed Susanna the cork to save from their special evening. They spent hours over that dinner and the food never stopped coming. Everyone talked non-stop with their hands and their warm smiles. They knew quite a bit of English and what Susanna didn't understand, Giovanni interpreted for her. There was absolutely no problem with communication. Mama apologized to her for not cooking. Can you imagine that? This wonderful Italian family completely accepted her.

As the sun sizzled behind the ancient Roman buildings, the stars came out but it was still very hot. Susanna held the back of her hair up off her neck to cool off. Patricia took a hair clip out of her own hair and handed it to Susanna. It was just a small gesture of kindness but one she would never forget. Sometime during dinner she thought to herself, "Here I am, a stranger from another country and now I am a part of this happy Italian family." Growing up, her own family never treated her with such love and acceptance. She thought, "Life just can't get any better than this."

Their joyous week together came to an end all too quickly. Giovanni drove Susanna back to the airport. It was much harder to part this time because they had become even closer. Standing at the gate, they held each other tight and cried. He promised to come to California in September when he had holiday time off. As her plane took off, she looked out the window at the panorama of Italy below and knew in her heart this would always be a place where she belonged. It felt like home to her.

CHAPTER EIGHTEEN

The Doctor Visit

Susanna was just Susan again without Giovanni by her side in California. She returned to the routine of work and looked forward to Giovanni's phone call every night. They missed each other so much. He asked her if she had made a doctor appointment. She reassured him that she had. He told her he was working a lot so he would have more money when he came to see her in September.

The night before her doctor appointment, Giovanni called to remind her about it. He sounded really worried about this. She told him not to worry. She said she was going the next day and was fine.

Doctor visits are always a nuisance but she had promised Giovanni she would go. She just wanted to get it over with. She drove to the hospital for her appointment. After removing her bra and putting on a hospital gown, she sat in the small exam room. As she waited, she thought of errands she needed to do before enjoying the rest of the beautiful day.

The young Doctor Dee entered the room and began examining her breasts. He felt a lump in her right breast. He told her not to worry. He said, "A lump doesn't mean you have cancer. Only about 1 in 12 lumps women get in their breasts are cancer." He then inserted a needle into the lump and discovered that it was solid. He left the room and returned with another doctor. This doctor also examined her breast. Both doctors then left the room together for a few minutes. When Dr. Dee returned, he repeated, "The lump we found is probably nothing to worry about. We want you to have an ultrasound, just to make sure."

"What a bother," she thought, "this is going to take more time." She put her blouse back on and walked down the hall to the room with the ultrasound machine. After changing into another hospital gown, she lay on the exam table as she was told. A nurse came in and slathered freezing cold gel all over her breast. This was not how she had planned to spend her day off!

Another doctor came in and attached wires to sticky dots. He stuck them all over her breast. He dimmed the lights and turned on the ultrasound machine. He began staring intently at the bright screen. This was an entirely new experience for her so Susan asked him if she could see too. He slowly turned the screen so she could see it from the table she was laying on. It was very clear to see. There was a solid black spot.

She got dressed and met Dr. Dee back in his office. He told her she had a tumor and he wanted to remove it right away. He explained that it was a simple procedure. She would be awake. He would numb the area, remove the tumor, give her a couple stitches and she would be on her way. She made an appointment for the following week and left. She wasn't worried, she was happy and life was grand. The hospital was near a shopping mall so she stopped there on her way home and bought some cute outfits to wear for Giovanni's visit.

Giovanni called that night. The first thing he said was, "What happened at your doctor appointment? Did he find the small ball in your breast?" She told him, "You were right, there is a small ball in my breast." She heard him suck in his breath. She cheerfully explained, "The doctor said not to worry. I've already made an appointment to have it taken out next week. I'll be fine." With that out of the way, they continued to have a happy conversation about more pleasant things.

CHAPTER NINETEEN

Three Worst Words

Susan returned to the hospital a week later. As promised, it was a simple procedure. It didn't take more than a half hour. The nurses and Dr. Dee came into the room dressed in bright yellow operating gowns. She laughed when she saw them. They looked like a bunch of baby chicks. She lay on the table and they injected a local anesthetic to numb the small area. It worked immediately. She was awake and alert. She talked to them while they were huddled over her chest. She happily told them, "I'm going to marry a man who lives in Rome!" "Congratulations!" was muffled behind their surgical masks.

They did an excisional biopsy, which means they took out the whole ball instead of just a slice of it. They put it in a clear glass of liquid. She told them she wanted to see what it looked like. They held the glass up so she could see it from her horizontal position. They told her the tumor was about 2.5 centimeters. It was about the size of a ball she used to play jacks with when she was a kid and it was pink. She thought, "That's a good thing. If it was cancer it would be purple or green or something weird looking, not a healthy looking pink ball."

Feeling just fine, she got dressed and went back into the doctor's office. He told her he would send the tumor to the lab to be tested and let her know the results in 10 days. She wasn't very sore. It was just a small incision about 1 inch long. Glad to have that over with, she left and enjoyed the rest of her day off. The weather was beautiful so she drove to the park near her house and took a short walk along the trail by the lake.

She really never gave it another thought until the tenth day. She called the hospital for the results. The woman who answered the phone said she couldn't tell her over the phone, she would have to come in and talk to the doctor. This made her a little nervous but not too worried.

The next day she was back, sitting in the little hospital room waiting for the doctor. Dr. Dee walked in a couple of minutes later. He gently put his hand on her shoulder and said the three worst words she would ever hear in her life, "You have cancer."

She felt disconnected, like it feels when driving through a thick fog, sounds are muffled and you can't see beyond the front of your car. Her brain refused to accept what her ears just heard. She couldn't talk, she couldn't think. Then, from somewhere in the fog, came her doctor's quiet voice again. "You have cancer, Susan. The lab results showed the

tumor had unclean edges. This means we didn't get it all."
"No! This isn't real!" she screamed inside her mind. Finally, for some unclear reason, she calmly told him, "No, I'm too young to have cancer, I'm only 43." With kind eyes, he looked into her unfocused eyes and quietly replied, "Young people get cancer too." The words slowly sank in.

It was all a blur after that. The doctor was saying strange foreign words, Infiltrating Carcinoma, Lumpectomy and Mastectomy. These were terrifying words she had never even heard of in 1992. He was telling her she would have to make choices. Her mind was numb. How could she possibly make choices when it was impossible to even think rationally? All she remembered was driving home alone on the freeway, sobbing during the entire half hour drive. So began Susan's very personal struggle with this frightening disease.

— CHAPTER TWENTY —

Tears

Her youngest son, Erin, who had just turned nineteen, was living at home with her. She decided as she pulled into her driveway that she didn't want him to know. She didn't want him to worry. That idea didn't work. As soon as she walked into the house, he asked her, "What's wrong?" in an alarmed voice. She burst into tears. She had a hard time even speaking the words. She finally said, "I have cancer." He put his strong arms around her and hugged her so tight. They stood in the kitchen like that for a long time until they finally stopped crying.

Giovanni called her from Rome a few hours later. She hated to give him such terrible news over the phone but had no choice. She could hear him crying through thousands of miles of telephone cables and knew she was the one who caused him such sorrow. She wanted so badly to promise him that everything would be ok but she couldn't. She didn't know.

The next day she dreaded making the phone calls but she had to call her Aunt and Uncle in southern California. She also had to call her best friend Cindy in Sacramento. She didn't want them to worry but felt she had to tell them the truth. They cried. It was so difficult to be the bearer of such shocking terrible news.

Her oldest son, Rick, had moved and she didn't have his new phone number. Someone located him because he called her in tears. He was so upset over the bad news.

Being a mom, this was so difficult. She had always been the one to dry her son's tears and tell them everything would be all right. It was just wrong to be the reason they were crying. She felt so guilty. She also felt ashamed because she was upsetting the people she loved.

CHAPTER TWENTY-ONE

Questions and Decisions

She had many questions for Dr. Dee on her next visit. He explained the three different procedures he could do. A Lumpectomy was a partial removal of the breast tissue around the tumor site. A Mastectomy was to remove the entire breast. The third was a mastectomy followed by reconstructive surgery. She chose to have a Lumpectomy. This decision probably had a lot to do with the fact that she was single and wanted to save as much of the breast as possible. She had been single for a long time and cared about her appearance. If she had been married for the past 20 years her decision may have been different.

Susan asked the doctor, "What did I do wrong? What did I do to cause this?" He told her they didn't know what caused breast cancer. He explained that our bodies have perfect round cells and that cancer cells are deformed and multiply quickly. They still don't know why our bodies all of a sudden start making these deformed cells. He said that, fortunately, she had a slow growing tumor. It had probably been growing there for about 7 years.

Giovanni made last minute plans to fly to California and be with Susan. She decided to delay her surgery for one month so they could spend some quality time together before she had to go into the hospital. Giovanni would be arriving in a few days. She had time at home alone to think about what the doctor had told her about the tumor.

First of all she was angry! She was pace-back-and-forth clenching her fists angry! She had been so careful to go to her doctor appointments every year and have breast exams. How could all of those doctors, every year for 7 years, have missed it? She had mammograms faithfully every year. Why didn't they see it on the X-rays? Why didn't her ex-boyfriend notice it? How could this be?

It was difficult to believe she had something as serious as cancer. She was in shock. She was young and had never had a life-threatening illness before. Her body hadn't given her any warning. She had no pain, fever or nausea, no symptoms to tell her something was going wrong inside.

After spending days being angry and trying to make rational sense of it all, she came to the realization that it was her own fault. She should have examined her own body. She should have noticed it. After she knew it was there, a lump next to her nipple, it was obvious. Giovanni found it the very second he touched her. It hit her then with full force! Giovanni was a miracle sent to her from God. If it weren't for him, she wouldn't have known until it was too late.

Susan had to go back to work and meet with her manager. She had to tell her she would need a medical leave of absence from work. Susan tried to be brave and professional but she was feeling so emotional. She started crying in her manager's private office when she had to say the word cancer. Her manager was very concerned and supportive. There was a mound of paperwork Susan needed to fill out for disability. After all the details were sorted out, her manager assured her that her job would be waiting for her after her recovery. Susan left without telling any of her co-workers good-bye. That would just be too hard to do.

CHAPTER TWENTY-TWO

Happy Days In Denial

When Giovanni walked through the customs gate, Susan felt such happiness to be with her love again. She also felt relief that she wouldn't have to go through her surgery alone. Giovanni hugged her tight and said, "I have been praying for you in St. Peter's every single day." Then, he just couldn't wait any longer. He slipped a diamond ring onto her finger, right there in the San Francisco airport. Susan was thrilled! She told him she didn't want to spend their month together being sad or worried. She wanted to feel happy and have fun again.

Well, have fun they did! She had been to his country but he had never been to hers. She drove him across the Bay Bridge to her cute little home. When they arrived, Giovanni exclaimed, "I didn't know you lived in a villa!" She never thought of herself owning a "villa" before.

When she took him into the big Safeway grocery store,

he was like a kid in a candy store. There are no big stores with everything under one roof in Italy. Together they bought lots of groceries so they could take turns cooking for each other. One night she took him out for pizza. It was so different from the pizza in Italy. He loved it. American pizza has a thick crust piled with toppings. Everyone around the table shares the same pizza, usually eating it with their hands. In Italy, the pizza is delicious with a very thin crust. It has only one topping covered with cheese. Everyone eats their own personal pizza with a knife and fork.

Giovanni and her son, Erin, really hit it off. Erin was full of questions about Italy. Giovanni told them wonderful stories about growing up in Italy. The way Giovanni sometimes arranged his words made Erin laugh. He was so happy for his mom. He could see how she glowed when she was with Giovanni. He totally approved. They were happy peaceful days at home.

Susan had a wonderful time showing Giovanni around on their mini vacations. They drove up to Lake Tahoe, Nevada. Giovanni thought it was the most beautiful place he had ever seen and Susan had to agree. Even though she loved the beauty of Italy, Lake Tahoe was still the most beautiful place on earth to her. They made love in their hotel room and enjoyed room service breakfast. Giovanni got to play a slot machine for the first time. He got lucky. He talked lovingly to his machine in Italian and the coins kept spilling out. He thought this was quite an easy way to make extra money. He wasn't there long enough to experience losing. They left to go enjoy a casino show and had a fabulous time.

They drove up the beautiful California coastline and stopped along the way to play on the beach. In the small town of Capitola they had lunch outside in the sunshine. They held hands as they leisurely walked along the boardwalk in Santa Cruz. Susan just couldn't get enough of that beautiful smile of his.

At Big Basin Park in the Santa Cruz Mountains they wandered along one of the trails, alone in the cool shade of the huge redwood trees. Their footsteps were muffled as they walked through the silent forest upon the cushion of pine needles. When they paused to look up, Giovanni was amazed at the massive size and height of these trees. There were pine trees in Italy but these giant redwoods were only found in California and southern Oregon. The sun was glinting bright rays through the dark green branches. Little fat squirrels were scampering around them. It was a positively glorious day! How could Susan possibly be so happy, knowing she had cancer? But she felt happier with Giovanni than she had ever been in her life.

The charming coastal town of Carmel was pleasantly warm in August with clear blue skies. They browsed through the many art galleries and discussed the differences between the paintings in the U.S. and the more religious paintings in Italy. Outside one of the shops, Giovanni grabbed Susan's hand and pulled her alongside the building. He put his arms around her and gave her a long loving kiss. A woman caught them as she was walking past. She just smiled and sighed, "Ah, I'm jealous." Susan smiled and thought to herself, "I'm the luckiest woman in the world to have this man."

CHAPTER TWENTY-THREE

Surgery

As Susan's surgery date, September 3, 1992 grew near, they had to return. Giovanni went with her to the doctor appointment. He asked questions. Dr. Dee explained that besides doing the lumpectomy, he wanted to remove 10 lymph nodes from under the arm to make sure the breast cancer cells hadn't spread through her bloodstream to other parts of her body.

During the entire month spent with Giovanni, Susan had managed to put the whole cancer thing out of her mind. She wasn't worried or scared. She just refused to think about it. It simply wasn't going to interfere with their happiness. However, the night before her surgery it hit her hard. She was scared to death. The only two times she had been in the hospital before were to have babies. Those were happy experiences. This was so different.

She finally had to face and accept the truth. She had a life threatening disease. The truth was, that every single person she had known who had cancer died within a year. The only person who had lived longer was her mom. She discovered she had cancer less than a year after Susan's husband died. The poor thing lived for 2 years before she died. Susan saw how much she suffered.

She called her Uncle Dick that night and told him she was scared. He talked to her for a long time and told her funny stories. He tried to get her mind off the surgery she was going to have to face the next morning. In bed that night, Giovanni held her. They talked long into the night. With only a couple hours of sleep they left for the hospital early the next morning. Susan's son, Erin, went with them.

Later that afternoon she woke up. The first thing she saw was Giovanni and Erin standing at the foot of her bed smiling. Still feeling the effects of the morphine, she asked, "Why are you guys smiling?" Here she was in a hospital bed with her chest wrapped in bulky bandages and they were grinning like fools. Giovanni happily told her, "The cancer cells didn't spread to any lymph nodes. They got all the cancer out!" As she drifted back to sleep, she vaguely remembered she didn't quite believe him because he wasn't a doctor.

Some time later she awoke with Dr. Dee standing by her bed. He confirmed what Giovanni told her was true. He told her she could spend the night or they could take her home. She wasn't in much pain then and wanted to go home. Erin and Giovanni had been walking all over the hospital looking around. When they came back into her room they both came to her bed and gave her kisses. They were so happy her operation was a success. Giovanni couldn't believe how nice the hospital was. He told her the amazing news that there were TVs in every room. Susan laughed!

CHAPTER TWENTY-FOUR

Facing The Future

Susan had to wear her robe home because it was too hard to get dressed. There was a hole under her arm with a clear tube coming out which extended down to her waist. At the end of the tube was a rubber bulb. This allowed fluids to drain. She could keep it hidden under her robe.

For the next week, after the strong drugs had worn off, she was in quite a bit of pain. They had removed a third of her breast as if cutting a wedge from a pie. She had a line of stitches running from her nipple to her underarm and up her underarm a few inches where they had removed the lymph nodes and cut muscle tissue. She couldn't move her arm because it hurt too much. It pulled on the stitches and tender muscles. She had instructions to walk her fingers up the wall, a little further every day, to stretch those muscles. It hurt.

Despite the pain, she was happy the outcome had been

a success. She knew she would feel better every day now. She was looking forward to her life being normal again. Giovanni and Erin cooked for her and took good care of her. She had made it. She could feel happy again. This whole horrible cancer episode was behind her.

A week later, Susan still couldn't use her arm to drive. Giovanni and Erin took her to the doctor for her appointment. While they stayed in the waiting room, she went in alone. A nurse removed the plastic tube from under her arm then sent her to the lab for a blood test. From here, she walked down the hall for a chest X-ray. She returned to meet with Dr. Dee with a big smile on her face, so looking forward to discussing good news.

He began by congratulating her for the successful surgery but her high spirits plummeted downhill from there. He started right in bombarding her with his words about months and months of treatments she would now have to go through. He told her she needed to begin Radiation treatments immediately. She would have to come to the hospital every day except weekends. These daily treatments would go on for many weeks. Then after that, she would most likely begin months of Chemotherapy.

She was shocked and confused. She told him, "I thought it was over. I thought you got it all!" He explained that he did get it all from the area around the tumor. She said, "But you said my lymph nodes were negative!" He told her he had removed and examined only 10 lymph nodes. He said there are between 30 and 60 lymph nodes under the arm. However, the lymph node evaluation doesn't give them a foolproof answer. Even with negative lymph nodes, 20-30 percent of breast cancers will have spread. This was devastating news to her. He recommended Radiation. He explained to her that this follow-up procedure was for her protection. She quickly learned that life as she had known it was over.

— CHAPTER TWENTY-FIVE —

The Hardest Thing

This was the nightmare she had feared. This was exactly what her mother had gone through before she died. Susan now knew she was going to die. She asked Dr. Dee what her chances of living were if she didn't have these treatments. He told her the medical studies showed that without follow-up treatments the chance of living longer than one year was in the 20 percent range. She understood then that she couldn't refuse treatments. At the same time she realized, with deep regret, that she couldn't have the normal life with Giovanni she so desperately wanted.

As Giovanni slept by her side that night, she lay there with her eyes open. Silent tears slid into her hair. She felt so helpless. Her life was spiraling downhill like water down the drain and there was nothing she could do about it. She knew what was ahead of her. This wonderful man next to her loved her more than she could ever have imagined. He wanted to spend the rest of his life with her. He loved her too much. She couldn't let him love her that much and watch her slowly die. As much as she loved him and wanted him with her, she just couldn't do that to him.

The next morning she took his hands in hers and quietly told him she wanted him to go back to Rome. It just about broke her heart. They argued all day. He gave her every reason why he should stay with her through this and she gave him every reason why he shouldn't. He told her he loved her so much. If she got sick he would take care of her. He didn't care if all her hair fell out. He would still love her. He wanted her to be his wife. This made her cry because she knew she probably wouldn't be alive to share a lifetime with him. She told him she loved him too, more than she ever thought she could love someone, but she stood her ground. She had to be strong. Making him leave was the hardest thing she ever had to do.

With a quick phone call, she changed his airline ticket and changed their future. She drove him to the San Francisco airport the next day. This was just too hard on both of them to delay it. She had to begin Radiation treatments immediately. They were very quiet while waiting for his departure. There was nothing left to say. With tears streaming down their cheeks, they just stood there silently holding each other. The last thing he said to her before turning to walk to the plane was, "I will pray for you my Susanna. I will love you forever."

She spent the rest of the day crying. This was the lowest point in her life. She loved this man beyond words and had to send him out of her life. She just kept telling herself over and over that it was better to end it now. It would be much harder for him to stay and watch her die.

Chapter Twenty-Six

Radiation

Susan began Radiation treatments the next day. Before her first treatment she met with the Radiologist. She asked him, "If I do this, what is the survival rate?" This time it was in the 50 percent range. It was still a 50-50 chance that she would live longer than one year but this gave her a small ray of hope. She had to try.

Radiation treatments changed Susan's lifestyle overnight. She now went to the hospital every day, Monday through Friday at noon. On her first day, she looked around for a dressing room to remove her shirt and bra. There wasn't one. They told her she had to leave modesty outside when she entered these doors. They marked a circle of dots around her breast then tattooed the dots with permanent ink so the area wouldn't have to be remarked every time. These dots made it an accurate target for the Radiation machine.

She was scared at first when she had to go into the room

by herself and lay topless under a machine the size of a dinosaur. The staff had to go outside the room and watch her on a video screen. She asked why she had to be in there alone. They told her they couldn't be exposed to that much radiation on a daily basis. She thought, "But, it's ok for me?" Susan had visions of becoming the Incredible Shrinking Woman.

These kind people became her new friends. She hung out with them every day. They joked around with her and made her smile. They told her right at the beginning she couldn't shave under that arm or wear deodorant. This news totally grossed her out! After a few weeks, there was one jovial black lady that made her burst out laughing when she exclaimed, "Ooh, honey. That's quite a bush you're growing there!"

The Radiation didn't hurt. It was rather like having an X-Ray at the dentist. In the beginning her nipple and breast just looked and felt like they were a little sunburned. Eventually though, after many weeks of treatments, they turned almost a black color and peeled twice.

The good news was that the radiation stopped her periods. The bad news was that she was thrown into menopause and couldn't take hormones to help. The type of breast cancer she had fed on hormones. This made her wonder if taking birth control pills for about 10 years caused her to have cancer. She asked her doctor. He said they didn't know. There was no proof. Hot flashes were the least of her worries though. The worst effect, by far, was how tired she became. Every day she drove home, collapsed on the couch and slept.

Fortunately, her son was working and didn't see her like this. It became very important to her that she should behave exactly as she used to before she got cancer. She didn't want anyone, including her son, to worry about her. So every afternoon after her nap she would get up and fix dinner for them. She would smile and never talk about her treatments. She wouldn't say the word cancer. Giovanni still called her from Rome every night. She always tried to sound positive over the phone. He told her he loved her as much as ever and wouldn't give up on them. As the weeks passed, she became more exhausted and weak. It was an awful feeling because she had always been an energetic person. Even though she slept every afternoon and every night, it didn't seem to help. She would wake up tired.

CHAPTER TWENTY-SEVEN

Hard Times

Being a single mom, there was little money left over to build up much of a savings. She had managed to save up a couple thousand dollars over the years but she had been unable to work for months now. Her savings was used up. Disability insurance finally kicked in. They sent her a check every week for $217.00. With $868.00 a month to live on, it was very hard. Fortunately, she had bought her little home years earlier and the house payments were low. She only had one credit card bill, which she had used for her Italy trip. She wrote to them about her situation and they agreed to minimum payments without interest. After she paid these bills plus her utilities and monthly car insurance payment, there was about $100.00 left for food for the entire month.

Even though Susan was very weak, she drove to the Social Security office and stood in line to try to get help from them. They gave her mountains of paperwork to fill out and mail in. This wasn't easy but she did it. A few weeks later she received a reply in the mail. They responded with, "The evidence indicates that your treatment has been successful and your condition is improving. Based on this evidence we have concluded that your condition will not prevent you from working for 12 months in a row." They would help her only if she was unable to work for more than 12 months. What was she supposed to do for money for food during those 12 months? Susan was so frustrated! She was supposed to be eating well and keeping herself free from stress. How could she do that when she was stressed out about not having enough money for food?

Throughout the previous years when people in her life needed help, Susan would give them a place to stay on her couch. She helped some of them out with a money loan to get them through their hard times. Well, now she was having a hard time and needed money. It was very hard for her to ask for help but she wrote letters to all the people who owed her money. She explained that she had cancer and couldn't work. She didn't ask for extra money, just the money back that she had lent them. She never heard back from any of them.

The doctors kept telling her she had to eat better to improve her strength. She had to do something. She began feeling desperate. She had to concentrate on herself now to get well. One night when her son came home, she sat down with him and explained that it was time for him to move out. She didn't have the money to support both of them anymore. He was 19 and had a job but she still felt horrible having to tell him. She had always been there for him since his dad died when he was only 3 years old. She couldn't do it any longer. It was time for him to learn to be on his own. She didn't know how much longer she would be around. He soon found a small apartment and moved out. Susan spent what she could to buy a few supplies he would need. It was the best she could do.

She was alone now. She wrote to her 2 half-sisters who lived in other states to tell them she had breast cancer. Their mom had cancer in other parts of her body but Susan didn't remember if she had breast cancer. She felt they should know since it could be hereditary. They didn't call. None of her old friends called. The only friend who called to see how she was doing was Cindy. She felt like she was being avoided like the plague. She tried to tell herself they were probably just uncomfortable and didn't know what to say to her about cancer.

Early one morning she awoke to the sound of raindrops on the roof. Wrapped in her fuzzy robe, she walked to the family room. She looked out the sliding glass doors into her back yard. The limbs of her bare fruit trees had silver drops sparkling on them as if they had become mystical creatures overnight. As she stood there looking at her apricot tree she thought of the 4th of July. The apricots were always sweet and plump with a tint of orange on them on the 4th. For years she always spent that weekend making homemade apricot jam. The uninvited thought crept into her mind, "Will I still be alive next 4th of July to make jam?"

Giovanni still called her every night. The day finally

came when she realized that she felt more depressed every time they hung up. It made her so sad wanting something she couldn't have. For so many months she had tried to act cheerful over the phone so he wouldn't worry. She kept telling him she was getting better. The truth was that she was actually feeling much worse. She was exhausted and felt like a rag doll. She didn't even feel like the same happy, hopeful person anymore that she was in Rome when they met.

CHAPTER TWENTY-EIGHT

Letting Go To Heal

Susan just couldn't do this anymore. After months of Radiation entering her body she was so weak. Her hope and strength had drifted away with the clouds. She experienced a level of despair she never thought possible. It was now just too difficult to keep up the act to Giovanni. Right or wrong, she made the decision. She had to lie to him to release him. She felt like she was wasting his time on a lost cause. He had such enthusiasm for life. It's what she loved the most about him. He had never let go of his faith that they would have a wonderful future together. She finally felt that it wasn't right to continue giving Giovanni hope.

The next time he called she said, "Giovanni, I have something to tell you. I've met someone else and I'm going to marry him." This was her final act to him to make him believe she was doing great and moving on with her life so he could move on with his. She had to let go of his hand, like he'd had to let go of hers when her train pulled away from the station. There were tears pouring down her face but he couldn't see them. It broke her heart to lie to him and hurt him so deeply.

Giovanni cried, "No, Susanna, you can't do this! I know how much you love me. We are the other half of each other. We belong together. I don't believe you!" She quietly replied, "You have to believe me." She hung up the phone quickly before her voice gave her away that she was crying. She didn't even tell him, "I love you." She didn't even tell him, "Goodbye." She loved Giovanni so much. She prayed she had made the right decision for both of them. She cried and cried until there were no tears left.

She felt like this was her last chance. It was time to focus entirely on her now, before there was nothing left of her. This felt very selfish. She had spent half of her life caring for her children. She cared about the feelings of the people in her life, especially Giovanni's. But, she had finally made the difficult decision. She needed to be completely alone now to grab on tight to that rope and concentrate on healing her body. She knew she had to change her way of thinking and begin a more positive attitude to get well.

At first she would lie down and relax, take deep breaths and imagine a bright white light filling her body with healing power. Who knows what makes the mind work? Soon the vision turned into a Pac Man game going on inside her body. Every day when she got home from her Radiation treatment she would lie on the couch and close her eyes. The white Pac Man would begin in her chest and travel all through her body gobbling up any black spots he came across. This game went on for months inside her. In the beginning she would concentrate really hard. After awhile it just happened naturally. She was totally alone at home now. God became her best friend. She would talk to him all the time and ask him to help her heal herself.

The day finally came when they happily announced it was her last Radiation treatment. She still had to go to the hospital once a week for blood tests but as the days passed and turned into weeks, Susan slowly began to feel a little stronger. Whenever sad thoughts of Giovanni and what they had together tried to enter her mind she would push them away. Thoughts of what his wonderful family must think of her tried to break in but she wouldn't let them. She couldn't. It was just way too painful.

— CHAPTER TWENTY-NINE —

"Smile"

Susan's Uncle Dick made her feel happy and loved. He had always been like a father to her. She flew to southern California to be with him. He met her at the airport and gave her a big hug just as he had done every summer since she was a child. They sat outside on the shady patio and talked the whole weekend. She told him about her fear of cancer and her sadness about not having Giovanni in her life. Uncle Dick understood the love she felt for Giovanni. He always understood her.

Uncle Dick played her an old song. Charlie Chaplin wrote the music. John Turner and Geoffrey Parsons wrote the lyrics. He told her it was written in the early 1950's during the time of the McCarthy trials. Charlie Chaplin was accused of being a Communist. Uncle Dick remembered that Charlie Chaplin denied the charge and it was never proven. This must have been a very difficult time for him because Charlie Chaplin left the country to live in Europe.

Uncle Dick said it was one of the most beautiful songs ever written. He confessed that he had played it during sad times in his own life. The words to this song went straight to her heart.

The title is "Smile".

> Smile, though your heart is aching
> Smile, even though it's breaking
> When there are clouds in the sky
> You'll get by
> If you smile through your fear and sorrow
> Smile and maybe tomorrow
> You'll see the sun come shining through
> For you
>
> Light up your face with gladness
> Hide every trace of sadness
> Although a tear may be ever so near
> That's the time you must keep on trying
> Smile, what's the use of crying
> You'll find that life is still worthwhile
> If you'll just
> Smile

Susan returned home and bought a tape with "Smile" on it. She played it many, many times. When she would start to feel down, the inspiring words from this song gave her hope for herself.

Giovanni called many times but Susan let the answering machine receive them. She didn't return his calls. It was so difficult to hear his voice and not rush to pick up the phone but she felt she had already hurt him too much. She still felt like a terrible person for lying to him. She hurt both of them but she had done what she felt she had to do. She had to accept that. She still didn't know if her Radiation and Pac-Man had missed any cancer cells hiding inside her somewhere. She felt it was best not to talk to him. She still wanted him to move on and have a happy life.

― CHAPTER THIRTY ―

The Fight Against Chemotherapy

Just when Susan was beginning to feel stronger she got a call from the hospital. They wanted her to come back in for another blood test and to see an Oncologist named Dr. Kay. She didn't even know what an Oncologist was. She thought he probably just wanted to check on her progress. She had really come to dread blood tests. She'd had so many her arm was bruised black and blue and was sore. She left the lab and walked over to the Oncologist's office. Patiently she waited to meet this new doctor.

As cool as a cucumber in his crisp white jacket, he walked in and introduced himself. The next words out of his mouth were, "We want you to start Chemotherapy treatments now." She was immediately upset. He had pushed her wrong button. She yelled, "No! I'm not going to let you poison me!" As the poor man stood there with his mouth open she stormed out of the room.

After all, what Susan knew of Chemotherapy was that you threw up everyday until you looked like a skeleton, all your hair fell out and you died. She felt like he had just given her the death penalty. By the time she got to her car she was shaking all over. She was so upset that he wanted to do this to her. She had given herself false hope, that because she didn't have cancer in the 10 lymph nodes, and because the doctor never mentioned Chemotherapy again, she wouldn't have to have it. She always swore after seeing what her mom went through that if she ever got cancer she would never ever have Chemotherapy.

The following week she had to go in for another blood test. Afterwards, the nurses shanghaied her back into Dr. Kay's office. "He just wants to talk to you", they said. This time he entered the exam room with another doctor. They were ganging up on her. They both started calmly telling her why they thought Chemotherapy would be the best thing for her. She screamed at both of them, "No, forget it! I won't let you poison me!" She slammed the door behind her right in their faces.

To avoid having Chemotherapy, Susan began reading everything she could get her hands on. She bought a book by Susan M. Love M.D. called Dr. Susan Love's Breast Book. It was an excellent book. It not only answered many questions about cancer procedures and treatments but also went into the emotional issues of having cancer. She found an article in a magazine about something fairly new called Tamoxifen, an estrogen blocker used in treating breast cancer. She made a copy of it and put it in her purse.

She received several phone calls on her answering machine from Dr. Kay but wouldn't return his calls. The lab called for more blood tests so she went to see them. When she walked out, Dr. Kay was waiting for her outside in the hall. She was so angry to see him she stomped behind him into his office to give him a piece of her mind and tell him to leave her alone. He calmly told her that the other doctor agreed with him about the Chemotherapy. She snapped back with, "You probably went to the same school!" He very patiently replied, "No, actually we went to different schools." He told her where both of them graduated. This doctor was really getting on her nerves. He just wouldn't give up. In a hysterical voice she screamed back at him, "You probably just want to poison me so you'll make more money!" He calmly replied, "No, actually the hospital will make less money if you have Chemotherapy treatments."

Susan pulled the paper out of her purse with the article about Tamoxifin and shoved it at him. He read it and told her he knew about it but thought it had too many bad side effects. He still believed Chemotherapy would be best for her. Frustrated at this point, Susan screeched, "I want my medical records. I'm getting another opinion!" He just calmly told her she was welcome to do that. She was such a total bitch to him and she knew it. She knew she was probably being irrational but she had been fighting this cancer for such a long time and didn't want to die now from being poisoned.

She marched straight down to the records department and left with a big manila envelope thick with her medical records. She would show him. She immediately made an appointment with 3 doctors at a hospital in San Francisco.

Dressed up in a pretty new outfit with her hair fixed and healthy-looking blush makeup on her cheeks, she confidently entered the San Francisco hospital. She was going to get the opinions of these new doctors. She thought, "Now I will have them on my side to back me up." An hour later she slunk back to her car with her tail between her legs. She was defeated. They had all agreed with Dr. Kay's decision to get Chemotherapy.

CHAPTER THIRTY-ONE

Giving In

This was the end of the road. There was no fight left in her. Susan went back to Dr. Kay and apologized for being such a bitch. He surprised her by telling her, "I respect you for what you did." She said, "You do?" He said, "Yes. Most of my patients just meekly accept whatever they are told without doing any research." He told her she was right, that Chemotherapy is a combination of poisons but low doses of these poisons could be beneficial in killing any cancer cells in her body that the surgery and Radiation could have missed.

Before agreeing, she asked Dr. Kay, "If I do this, what is the survival rate?" This time the number was in the high 70 percent range of living longer than one year. She began to feel very hopeful but then remembered her mother. She had probably been told the same thing. Susan talked to Dr. Kay then. She told him all about her mom. She explained to him that this was the reason she was so afraid of Chemotherapy. It was the final stage before death.

He then understood her fear. He said in1981, when her mom died of cancer, that it was still the dark ages of cancer research. He told her they had come so far since then. He said in a five-year study, a high percentage of cancer patients survived now. She heard him say five years and exclaimed, "Five years! I want to live longer than five years!" He clarified his statement by saying, "We've only done a five-year study. No one knows how long you'll live after that. You might get run over by a truck!" Susan finally laughed again. She certainly didn't feel good about having Chemotherapy but she accepted it.

Before starting Chemotherapy, Susan drove to Sacramento to spend the weekend with her friend Cindy. She felt like this might be their last girlfriend weekend together. As soon as she walked into Cindy's apartment she saw a huge pile of cancer brochures on her coffee table. Cindy wanted knowledge to be able to talk to her friend about cancer. That's the kind of friend she was. Susan wouldn't talk about it at all. She just kept smiling, pretending to be the same person she used to be on their girlfriend weekends. Cindy didn't push her.

After a fun weekend of laughing and shopping it was time to leave. Cindy hugged her and Susan burst into tears. Cindy exclaimed, "Thank God! I was beginning to think you weren't human!" Susan couldn't help but laugh. That old sense of humor Cindy always had is what Susan loved best about her friend. Before she left, Susan told Cindy she was beginning Chemotherapy the following week.

During that week, Susan read a book called "Chemotherapy and You" put out by the U.S. Department of Health and Human Resources. It had information about relaxation, self-hypnosis and imagery. She was on the right track. She was already doing this. She read that she should open the lines of communication. She should share feelings, desires and worries about Chemotherapy. She wanted to, she knew it would probably make her feel less tense about it, but she couldn't. She was terrified but it wouldn't change anything to talk to her Aunt and Uncle, her sons, or her friend Cindy. She still had to go through it alone. Besides, they had never had cancer. They couldn't understand what she was feeling.

She wished she could talk to someone who had been through Chemotherapy. There were so many scary unknowns buzzing around in her head. She wanted to ask questions like, "Did it burn? How did it make you feel?" She couldn't even ask her doctors these questions. They had never been through it themselves. She wanted to ask someone even dumb questions like, "Did you lose your eyebrows? Could you finally stop shaving your legs? Did your hair ever grow back?" But she didn't know anyone who had gone through Chemotherapy and lived to talk about it. There weren't any support groups that she could find. There was just no one to turn to or talk to at that time. She had to keep quiet and bury her unanswered questions and fears deep inside.

— CHAPTER THIRTY-TWO —

Terrified

The most terrifying day of Susan's life was her first day of Chemotherapy. Dr. Kay met her in his office first. She couldn't stop shaking and crying no matter how hard she tried. He called in the anesthesiologist to talk to her and try to calm her down. Dr. Kay told him about her experience with her mom. The anesthesiologist assured her that this wasn't a death sentence. He promised that he would do everything to make her well and keep her from being too nauseated. All she could do was manage to nod her head.

They led her into a room with a recliner chair and a TV. It felt to her like she was walking into the death chamber. They inserted a needle into her arm and she watched the poison flowing through the tube into her body. There was nothing she could do but sit there with the I.V. in her arm for the next hour. It was torture, more mental than physical, knowing she was being poisoned. It didn't burn. It felt cold. She just sat there in silence with tears streaming down her cheeks.

That night, the anesthesiologist called her at home to see how she was feeling. It was nice to know that he cared. She told him her stomach was upset but probably from nerves and from crying all day. There was no vomiting. She had been through quite an ordeal that day and had survived her first Chemotherapy treatment. She thanked God and slept.

Somehow, she endured 5 more of these treatments over the next 6 months. Right after the treatments she would feel a little nauseated and weak for the next few days and would stay in bed but then it would pass. She didn't lose all her hair. It just became very thin and seemed to turn white overnight. At this point she didn't much care. Her eyebrows and eyelashes stayed put and unfortunately she still had to shave her legs. The vein in her arm finally collapsed after so much use. They had to start putting the needle in her hand which was much more painful. They also took blood tests every time she went in. She had so many bruises.

Susan lost her appetite and wasn't eating as much but every time she went to the hospital she had gained another few pounds. She began to look bloated all over. She couldn't understand this and asked Dr. Kay about it. He told her it was a side effect from the Chemotherapy drugs. He told her not to worry, that she would lose it when her treatment was over.

The poison gave her really creepy nightmares. Over and over she dreamed that she had killed someone. She had their body stuffed in a big Hefty bag. She felt no remorse about killing them. Her only concern was what to do with this big Hefty bag. Night after night in her dreams, she would be dragging this bag all over, trying to find a bush to bury it next to. What a weird dream! She analyzed it herself. She must have been getting rid of the cancer every night by taking it out and burying it. She wondered if other Chemotherapy patients had nightmares.

Her aunt and uncle were worried about her being alone through her treatments. They begged her to come live with them. She was tempted. It would have been easier to let them take care of her. But, she decided against it because she needed to be close to the hospital. One weekend between treatments, when she thought she could handle it, she flew to see them. She wanted to put their minds at ease. She wanted them to see for themselves that she was fine so they would quit worrying. Her uncle paid for her ticket. He was taking it especially hard. Susan's mom was his only sister. Susan thought she was doing fine during the hour flight and the drive to their home. Unfortunately, as soon as she arrived she felt dizzy and nauseated. She had to spend the day in bed and wished she had never come. They became even more worried seeing her in bed. It turned out to be a bad idea. The trip was made too soon before her body was ready.

It may be hard to believe, but Susan actually had good days during those 6 months. She would sit out in her backyard with the sun shining and the birds singing. She felt happy just to be alive. She was thankful for these beautiful days. She used every ounce of her energy to get well. Thoughts of Giovanni kept getting buried deeper and deeper as she did everything she could possibly do to survive.

CHAPTER THIRTY-THREE

A Survivor!

At the end of 11 long hard months of enduring surgery, radiation, chemotherapy and a million blood tests, Susan went back to see Dr. Kay. He walked into his office where she sat waiting. With a beaming smile on his face, he handed her a piece of paper. She didn't know what it was and began reading it.

She read…

Hospital-Certificate of Achievement

This is to recognize Susan, who has completed 6 months of Chemotherapy. She has also suffered nausea, fatigue, hair loss and many bruises, but her bravery is hereby declared.

Signed:
Dr. Kay, the anesthesiologist and the pharmacist.

She looked into his eyes, feeling disbelief. She asked him, "Am I done? Is it over?"

He replied, "It's over."

She jumped up and hugged Dr. Kay. She was laughing and crying at the same time. He said he thought she would appreciate the certificate. She told him that he and everyone else at the hospital had done an excellent job. She couldn't have asked for better care. All of them working together had saved her and made her well. She asked him what her chances of living longer than one year were now. He told her, "You are now in the high 90 percent range." She wanted to hear 100 percent but was thrilled to be in the high 90's.

He said she could return to work. She never knew she could be so happy to go to work. After such a long time, it was hard for her to believe at first that it was finally over. He told her she would need to have blood tests and mammograms every 3 months, then every 6 months, finally once a year like normal people. She thanked him with all her heart for not giving up on her. It was really over. She had sacrificed a lot but she was a survivor.

She had a long talk with God that night. She thanked him for being by her side and holding her hand through it all. She thanked him for the miracle he had given her. She thanked him for her life.

CHAPTER THIRTY-FOUR

Starting Over

Susan returned to her job with the airlines. It felt so foreign and strange to be there at first. She had been gone almost a year. The job was exactly the same as it was when she left but she was different. After everything she had been through, she would never be the same again. Her co-workers welcomed her back. She hadn't told any of them that she had cancer but she suspected they knew. She could see the shock on some of their faces when they looked at her thin white hair. She couldn't color it before she went back to work. After being soaked with so many chemicals, her doctor wanted her to wait a couple of months before she poured more on her head.

After about 8 weeks her hair had grown back and was thicker than it was before. She used to have straight hair. Her new hair grew in wavy and pretty. She just couldn't get used to the white color. She didn't look like her old self.

Finally, she went to the drugstore and bought the same reddish blond hair color she used to have. After gooping it on and washing her hair, she removed the towel and looked in the mirror. It was a thrill to see her old self again smiling back at her.

When she got her first paycheck she let out a whoop! It wasn't a lot of money but it was a whole lot more than she'd been trying to live on for so long. With paychecks coming in again, she got her credit card paid off and started a savings account. She lost the puffy weight she had gained. She bought fresh fruits and green vegetables every week and cut way back on fatty foods. It felt so very good to have enough money to buy lots of good healthy food! She realized how important and exciting the little things in life were to her now.

Eventually she made new friends and even started dating again but never to an intimate level. She thought, "No man will ever want me." She wore a padded bra. She wouldn't have to feel embarrassed because no one would know what was hidden inside. She didn't tell anyone she was a cancer survivor. She never talked about cancer.

She felt guilty, a sense that she had done something wrong. She felt ashamed because she had pushed away those she loved. She felt different from other people. Because she didn't have therapy or a support group to work through these feelings, they just stayed inside her. She couldn't rationalize why she had these feelings, she just did. The only way for her to deal with these feelings, her scary cancer memories and her past painful memories of Giovanni, which were all intertwined like a ball of snakes, was to put them all out of her mind and pretend they never happened.

A year later, she met Gerry and knew he was different from the other men she'd been dating. They had a lot in common and enjoyed many of the same things. He had done a little traveling and wanted to do more. This was important to her. They had a great time as they got to know one another and fell in love. They went to plays and wonderful restaurants in San Francisco. He took her to Monterey with him on his scuba diving trips. They went hiking in Yosemite.

One of the things that attracted her to him was that he was independent. He had survived 2 bad marriages. He had been a single parent too and was doing just fine on his own. She felt in her heart that if they became more involved, he would be able to carry on without her if her cancer returned and she died.

It was their first ski weekend together in the mountains. Dinner was over and it was bedtime. It was time to tell him the truth. She couldn't put it off any longer. She had to tell him she was a cancer survivor. He needed to know what he was getting into before it went any further. She wanted to give him the chance to change his mind about being with her.

Gerry would be the first person to see her deformed breast and she was quite nervous. He was standing across the bedroom with his back to her when she said, "I have scars from breast cancer surgery. I finished my treatments a year ago." Without turning around, he told her something personal about himself. He said, "I have psoriasis." He didn't ask her any questions about the cancer. To her relief, it didn't seem to bother him.

They continued dating for the next 18 months. The subject of cancer was never brought up again after their first night together. Gerry never asked how she discovered she had cancer. He didn't ask any questions at all. This was fine with her because she didn't want to talk about it anyway. They had both been single for quite a few years. They never asked each other about past relationships. It didn't matter.

On a crisp March evening in 1995 at the Ahwahnee Hotel in Yosemite, Gerry asked Susan to marry him. She was so surprised she couldn't even speak. He said, "Say yes so I can give this to you." He held out a sparkling diamond ring. She finally found her voice and said, "Yes!" Less than 3 months later they got married at their friend's home in the mountains of Lake Tahoe, Nevada. The ceremony took place outdoors under the towering pines with their 3 grown children gathered around them. They toasted to their future as their international flight took off. They spent their marvelous honeymoon in England and Scotland!

The first 4 years of their marriage were very busy. They sold both of their homes and bought a home together. Susan was back in Alameda where her first husband used to play baseball on the weekends with members of the Oakland Raiders. It was really a strangely familiar feeling when a Raider named Tim Brown bought the house next door.

Susan and Gerry bought a half-acre lot in the mountains of Incline Village, Nevada for their retirement. Both of them were busy with full time jobs, at times working different shifts.

She secretly examined her breasts for lumps but never discovered any. She didn't think about cancer except once a year when she had to go in for a mammogram. After she had her mammogram she would find herself being on edge and irritable, afraid that the mammogram might show another tumor. When the test results arrived in the mail saying the mammogram was normal, she would breathe a huge sigh of relief. She would not have to think about it again until the following year. She never told her husband of her secret fears. She never told anyone.

— CHAPTER THIRTY-FIVE —

Adventure Of A Lifetime

Gerry enjoyed traveling almost as much as Susan. They took many fun vacations from work together. Their travels took them to ancient Greece, through the rain forests of Costa Rica, down the fascinating Amazon River in Peru and up the Eiffel Tower in Paris. Susan told Gerry she had always dreamed of taking time off and traveling all around Europe.

Her dream came true in April 1999. They quit their jobs, sold the house and cars and put their stuff in storage. There were definitely moments when she thought she must be crazy to give up everything and just take off for the unknown. She also knew that we don't know how long we will have to live. We have to try to make all our dreams come true and never give up trying.

With just 3 suitcases each and no definite plans beyond flying to the Frankfurt airport, they took off into the friendly skies. For the next 18 months they had their adventure of a lifetime. They drove everywhere and did everything their hearts desired. They spent leisurely time living in every country in Europe. It was an incredible experience. Susan was so happy she took this chance. She loved living in Europe. It was a dream, come true. They found inexpensive places to stay so the money they made from their house sale would last. They rented Hertz cars and paid cash for everything. It was exhilarating to have no bills and no responsibilities. They had a good marriage and made many great memories together.

From Frankfurt, Germany, they drove to Italy to begin their adventure. They rented an apartment in a small village just outside of Rome. It was out in the country surrounded by fields of glorious red poppies. Susan called her aunt from a pay phone one afternoon and was devastated to hear that her Uncle Dick had just passed away. He had always been her hero. She couldn't imagine her life without him. They had flown to see her Aunt and Uncle before they left for Europe just 6 weeks earlier. The last thing her Uncle Dick said to her was, "When I'm feeling better, we'll go to Italy to visit you." That evening Susan sat alone on their porch swing in the yard. Her eyes were blurry with tears as she looked out at the fields and thought about Uncle Dick. There were so many special memories. Just then, the sky became bright red. It was the most incredible sunset she had ever seen. She felt her Uncle Dick's presence and knew he had kept his word. He came to Italy to let her know he loved her one last time.

Susan never thought about Giovanni, not even while she was living in Italy for 3 months. To think of Giovanni would mean she would also have to think about the nightmare of having cancer. She wouldn't do it. She couldn't do it. Those old memories were buried deep inside now.

When they were in Siena, Italy, they went to the Palio di Siena. Susan had wanted to return for the famous horse race ever since her first visit to Siena. Another one of her dreams came true. She got to be stuffed in the middle of Il Campo square with all the locals and tourists. The contrada enthusiasm was exciting. The parades and elaborate costumes were incredible.

One day they went to a laundromat in Sorrento Italy. Here they met a fun couple named Rob and Evelyne who were vacationing. As they folded underwear together they laughed as they told stories about their travels. Rob and Evelyne loved to travel too. They learned that Rob and Evelyne used to live in Incline Village. What a small world. That's where their lot was. Rob and Evelyne had recently moved down the mountain but only lived about an hour away. For the next 17 months they kept in touch with E-mails.

Susan and Gerry had planned to move to Incline Village to build a home on their lot when their European adventure was over. About 2 months before their return, Susan began to have trouble falling asleep. She would toss and turn in bed thinking about how she wanted the design for their mountain home. Gerry finally went to an art store and bought her a large pad, pencils and a ruler so he could get some sleep. She would happily sit still in bed every night now, engrossed with sketching and erasing over and over while Gerry slept peacefully. She finally got the house designed just the way she wanted it before their departure date.

At the end of their adventure, Susan was sad to leave Europe. She loved it so much. The only things she missed in the United States were her sons, grandchildren, shopping with Cindy and Fig Newtons. She tried to convince Gerry to stay. She suggested they could sell their lot and build a little house in the French or Italian countryside. She came up with another idea. They could rent a chalet in Switzerland and have their kids visit them there. She tried hard to talk Gerry into staying but he wouldn't go for any of her ideas.

After staying to see the awesome Passion Play in Oberammergau, Germany, they flew back to the United States in October of 2000. Germany had been so lush and green. California was so dry and brown.

Fortunately they didn't stay in California. They rented a car and drove up to Lake Tahoe. Arriving with just their 6 suitcases full of worn out clothes, they were ready to start over and begin the next phase of their lives in the beautiful mountains of Nevada.

As soon as they arrived in Incline Village, they visited a local rental agency. They immediately moved into a temporary furnished condo. It only took 5 minutes to move in. They didn't have anything. They drove down the mountain into Reno and quickly bought a 4-wheel drive vehicle. They weren't picky about choosing it. They just needed something to drive in the mountains. It would be snowing soon. They were able to do a one-way rental with Hertz and dropped their car off while they were in Reno. It was all much easier than they thought it would be.

A week later they got lucky and found a furnished condo for sale. It was furnished in the 70's but it was perfect for them because all of their belongings were still in storage in California. The condo was only about a mile from their lot so they would be close to the building site.

To spend less money, they decided to be the contractors. They had no experience but figured they would learn as they went along. They immediately met with an architect to get started on their new house. Susan gave him her sketches to be put into proper dimensions. They hired local excavators, engineers, builders, electricians, plumbers and painters and the work began.

What was left in their savings, they used to begin the work. They would get a construction loan. Surprise! Surprise! The first 2 lenders turned them down because they didn't have jobs. They couldn't stop the work. They already had too much money into it. With faith that they could do it, they continued on with the building. They wouldn't give up. Were they really crazy? They finally got a loan on their third try. It didn't take long to be back in debt again but they were making their next dream come true, to build a house in the mountains of Lake Tahoe!

They were very busy during the building. Gerry spent every day up at their lot supervising and helping with the construction. Susan spent most days shopping for lighting, toilets, windows, appliances and door handles. The shopping list went on and on.

~ CHAPTER THIRTY-SIX ~

Acceptance At Lake Tahoe

On a warm summer evening in 2002 Susan and Gerry went for a walk to enjoy the pristine mountain scenery and beautiful weather. As they walked by the high school they noticed parked cars along the street. There was some event going on out on the track. They wandered back and saw a banner that read, "Relay for Life". They had never heard of this. They asked the woman sitting at a table about it. She told them it was an event to raise money for the American Cancer Society for cancer research. They thought this was a good cause so they walked in.

If Susan had known what was going to occur in the next few minutes she would have turned and made a run for it. The woman had purple t-shirts with a Relay for Life logo on the front. She asked if they would like to buy them to wear for the event. "Sure!" they said. She then asked, "Are you survivors or supporters?" Gerry said, "Both."

The next thing she knew, Susan was wearing a purple t-shirt with the words YOU CAN BEAT CANCER, I'M LIVING PROOF in big bold letters across her back for the world to see. She wanted to become invisible. She didn't want anyone to know her secret. As she turned to leave, this sweet lady said, "Please stay." Now that she knew Susan was a cancer survivor, she said, "Survivor's t-shirts are free. You also get a free dinner!" Since they were still fairly new to this area, Susan finally said, "Oh well, I don't know anyone here anyway."

This lady was also selling white paper bags called Luminarias. When they asked her about these, she told them, "You can write the name of a cancer survivor or the name of someone who lost their life to cancer on the bag. We fill them with sand and a candle. The entire track will be lined with the Luminarias. At sunset, we light the candles to remember and honor the cancer victims. Everyone walks around the track at their own pace." Susan bought one and wrote her mom's name on it. All they had to do now was go for a walk around the track. That was fine. They were out for a walk anyway.

There was a stage set up in front of the bleachers. Every time they walked around the track they would pause by the stage to watch the entertainment. There were singers, dancers, clowns and even a magician. Susan and Gerry were enjoying themselves when an announcer came on stage and said it was time for the Survivor Walk. They didn't know what this was. Susan wanted to go sit on the bleachers but Gerry talked her into staying on the track for the walk.

Susan had assumed that all the people here were just attending to raise money for cancer research and to see the entertainment. She was shocked to see so many people out on the track with the words YOU CAN BEAT CANCER, I'M LIVING PROOF on the backs of their shirts! It was almost her 10-year anniversary of being cancer free. She had kept this secret locked inside for all those years. Suddenly, she found herself surrounded by many others who had been through the same thing she had been through. They all looked happy. They held up a "Survivor" banner and began walking around the track with it. Susan walked in the middle of the group so she wouldn't be noticed.

The most amazing thing happened next. People were cheering and clapping for them as they walked past. Susan looked into their faces and they were smiling. She saw no looks of sadness or sympathy, only of happiness, respect and encouragement! These kind people of this small village called Incline accepted her for what she was, a cancer survivor. There are no words to express how deeply Susan felt at that moment.

As the sun began to set and the sky above turned a deep shade of lavender, the volunteers respectfully lined the track with hundreds of Luminaria bags and lit the candles one-by-one. The crowd gathered around the stage. The announcer began to say a prayer and a quiet peace settled over the mountains. His prayer was for the many people who had lost their lives to cancer, for those who survived, and for those who were currently fighting the disease. Susan thought of her poor mom who had fought so hard and died. She thanked God for how fortunate she had been to have had the disease at a time of advanced cancer research. She had been able to survive.

She listened to the announcer's words as she gazed around the track, glowing with hundreds of luminary bags, all with different names. The dam inside her cracked and crumbled. The tears flowed down her face and wouldn't stop. This very emotional moment was a huge release of the secret pain she had been holding inside for so many years.

This unexpected event in her life made such a huge impact on her, she volunteered to help the following year. They had a lot of fun. It helped Susan to be able to do something. She had felt so helpless when she had the disease. This was a way of fighting back. She learned how much work the volunteers put into the American Cancer Society Relay for Life. It felt so good to be able to help raise money for a cure. It was worth the effort for all the volunteers.

Susan also learned that the money raised by Relay for Life events all over the United States every year has helped enormously. It is the largest source of private, not-for-profit, cancer research funds in the United States, second only to the federal government in total dollars spent. In 2004 the Society spent nearly $131 million in research.

Cancer research has progressed by leaps and bounds just in the past 24 years since her mom died from this disease. Cancer isn't always a death sentence anymore. There is hope now. If caught early, there are a large percentage of survivors.

Susan and Gerry made many new friends through the

Relay for Life, the guys building their new house and from a club called Incliners. She wasn't shy about asking for donations for the Relay for Life. People gradually learned she was involved because she was a cancer survivor. Once in awhile someone would ask, "How did you discover you had cancer?" She wasn't ready to reveal her story yet so she would just tell them she discovered it herself.

Susan bought a Hallmark card for Dr. Kay for her 10-year Anniversary of being cancer free. She called the hospital in California to make sure he still worked there. He was still there. The card read-

"CONGRATULATIONS!"

She wrote,

Dr. Kay,

I hope you remember me. I'm the one who worked for the airline and fought with you so much about having Chemo. I just wanted you to know that it's my 10-year anniversary of being cancer free. Congratulations! You won the battle and I won the war!

Thank you for not giving up on me,

Susan

CHAPTER THIRTY-SEVEN

Magic In The Air

It was a busy 3 years since they moved to Incline Village but the house finally got finished and they moved into their beautiful new mountain castle. During these 3 years they saw Rob and Evelyne, the couple they met in the laundromat in Sorrento, Italy. They got together about once a month for dinner and became much more than good friends. There was a spiritual connection between them. They would talk and laugh long into the night. Dinner was never enough time together.

They all loved to travel and would spend hours discussing different countries, the people, the culture and the beauty in the world. They shared personal problems about families. They shared their dreams about what they wanted to do with the rest of their lives. The only thing Susan never shared was that she had survived cancer. In the back of her mind she was afraid it might spoil their wonderful relationship somehow if they knew she was different.

One lovely summer afternoon they had lunch with Rob and Evelyne in the tiny historical town of Truckee. From here they drove the short distance to Donner Lake to see an outdoor Glen Yarborough concert. It was one of those perfect warm summer evenings in the mountains. They sat in lawn chairs on the green grass and watched the sky turn from bright blue to bright orange to pale pink as the sun set over the clear still water in the lake. Towering pines surrounded the area like a wreath and filled the air with their fresh pine scent. They could hear the ducks out on the lake telling each other goodnight.

Perhaps it was the clear voice of Glen Yarborough as the touching words in his songs swirled around the trees like a mist or perhaps there was a bit of magic in the air that evening. When he took a break, Evelyne and Susan were teary eyed and emotional. They began talking about their personal feelings.

Maybe it was just the right time. Susan finally told her dear friend that she was a cancer survivor. Evelyne was such a caring person that she began asking Susan questions. When she asked her how she discovered she had cancer, the whole story came pouring out. Susan had enough trust in Evelyne to tell her all about Giovanni and the love they had for one another. Evelyne also asked about her visual memories of Italy, the sounds and the scents. Evelyne was a grand lady. In her wonderful way she got Susan to remember every detail.

They were both crying by the end of the story. Evelyne

hugged Susan. She thanked her for sharing her story and told her that she loved her more than ever. She asked Susan if she had called Giovanni at the end of her 11 months of treatments. Susan quietly told her, "No, I felt I had already hurt him too much to call him again."

After a few quiet moments Evelyne suddenly clapped her hands together and exclaimed, "You have to write a book about this!" Susan responded with a definite, "No!"

Evelyne asked her, "Why? It's a beautiful story." Susan told her, "Because Gerry doesn't even know the story about Giovanni. We never talked about it. Now that we've been married for so long, I don't feel right writing a story about my past love."

This grand lady with all her infinite wisdom surprised Susan by shouting, "Oh Pishaw! Why would Gerry mind? This all happened before you even knew him." She pleaded with Susan, "It's a beautiful story that needs to be told." Susan again said, "No."

Evelyne quietly asked her one question, "If it saved one person's life, would you do it?"

Without hesitating, Susan quietly answered, "Yes."

CHAPTER THIRTY-EIGHT

The Truth

I am Susan. I am a cancer survivor. Every word of my story is true. It was so emotionally difficult for me to write my story. To do it, I had to unbury and revisit the terrifying and heartbreaking memories that I had tried so hard to push deep down inside me. The only way I could get through it was to write as if it happened to someone else.

This is my 13-year anniversary of being cancer free. I can finally face the nightmare memories of the battle I went through and be thankful that I am still alive. I can finally remember Giovanni and the incredible love we shared. How could I have buried him along with my pain and fear? I will never forget him. How could I? He saved my life.

Kind people who have never been through the daily battle with cancer refer to those who have with words like courage and bravery. I don't think of myself as being coura-geous or brave. I did what I had to do so I could live. I just kept taking one step after the other. I was faced with many decisions. I had to make these very emotional decisions by myself. None of us ever knows for sure if we've made the right decisions in life. All any of us can do is the best we can at the time.

I still believe I made the right decision about my husband, Gerry. He has been a very strong and independent man throughout our years of marriage.

I have accepted the fact that with breast cancer, unlike some other cancers, 5 years without a recurrence doesn't mean I'm cured. Because it's a slow growing cancer, it can spread to another part of my body and go undetected for even 20 years. The more years I go without a recurrence, the less likely there is to be one. This is something I can live with.

My life will never be the same as it was before. The fears come back occasionally. Just when I stop thinking about cancer, something will pop up in an article or on the news about a risk factor or a new treatment, and it all comes back to me. But my fears are a part of my life, not the center of it anymore.

I recently had dinner with a friend. She is a well-educated bright lady. I told her I was writing a book about my discovery of breast cancer and asked her if she did self-breast exams at home. She replied, "No, I have a mammogram every year. I let the doctor take care of that." I told her that I also had breast exams by doctors every year and they never felt the cancer tumor I had in my breast. When I told her it never showed on any of my mammograms she was shocked! This just confirmed to me that I needed to write this book.

CHAPTER THIRTY-NINE

Get To Know Your Breasts!

I am not an expert about breast cancer. I don't claim to have the answers. All I can tell you is what I learned from this. Get to know your breasts! Do your own breast exams frequently. You don't have to wait until a certain day of the month and do it in the shower with soapy hands. You might forget the day and not get around to it.

Get into the habit of self breast exams while you're sitting on the couch watching TV in your robe at night. Take a good look at yourself in the mirror after your shower. Become very familiar with your breasts.

Remember, doctors examine many, many people every day. They are just human. They can miss things. Don't put your complete trust in someone else. They're your breasts. Be in charge of them. If you get to know your breasts very well, you will notice if something feels different. You will feel or see a lump.

Don't make the same mistake I did. I paid no attention to my breasts. I never looked at them. I never felt them. I never even thought about them.

Don't be distressed that if you go to the doctor, you may have to have mutilating surgery, that you will be deformed and no longer sexy. Dealing with these emotions is better than dealing with death.

Ask your partner to pay attention. I've heard that many women discovered they had breast cancer because their partner felt a lump.

Don't put off seeing your doctor until you can afford it. Saving your life by going to the doctor is more important than any bills that are due. Taking care of the bills can be done later.

If you're the type of woman who prefers "not to know," get over it. This way of thinking is just plain stupid. Early detection is the key to saving your life!

Pay attention to the news and articles. Chances are, you may never get breast cancer but it's a good idea to keep informed. If you're interested, read Dr. Susan Love's Breast Book. I'm not promoting it. I don't even know her. All I know is that I got so much information from this book that I never knew before. The more knowledge you have, the better.

If you do notice a lump or an area that doesn't look or feel quite right, don't ignore it. Don't think it will just go away if you ignore it. Go the doctor immediately. Insist they take tests.

Don't feel like you've got something awful and you will

have to undergo major surgery. Probably you won't. Chances are it's not cancer.

Go to the doctor immediately if you think you might possibly have a lump. Don't feel embarrassed because he might think you're making a big deal out of nothing.

Make sure to get yearly mammograms. This is important! Just because my tumor didn't show up then, doesn't mean it doesn't work. Mammograms have detected tumors in many women and saved their lives. I still get stressed out every year until I receive my normal mammogram results. I suppose I always will but I'll never stop getting them every year.

If you do get breast cancer, let the doctors do everything that the best of modern medicine and current knowledge provides. They know what they're doing. It's OK to get a second opinion. The doctor's feelings won't be hurt.

Try healing visualization. Fill yourself with white healing light and play Pac-Man in your body. I can't say for sure if it helped me but I believe it did.

Fear of cancer is an overwhelming feeling. Don't keep your fears and feelings hidden inside. Don't make the same mistake as I did. Call the American Cancer Society right away for help. There are many cancer support groups now. Ask your doctors. They can probably help with information about cancer support groups also. Make however many calls it takes to find a support group that you feel comfortable with.

Most importantly, I truly believe the reason I have been cancer free for 13 years is because I thank God every single night for my healthy body and for keeping me cancer free.

— CHAPTER FORTY —

Are There Angels In Italy?

There's not a doubt in my mind. I didn't think about it at the time but looking back, it's crystal clear to me. It all began when God gave me the visions of the fountain in Rome.

Father Boyle came next. Never before, or after, in my 10 years working at the airline did a priest ever invite me to spend the night at the Vatican. This angel gave me the confidence to travel to Italy alone.

Before I got on the train, I told myself, "If I feel lonely or uncomfortable or lost, all I have to do is turn around and go back home." My next 3 angels were Ricardo, Edward and Frank, on the train from Frankfurt to Italy. They were so friendly and kind that I didn't feel uncomfortable.

My next angel was dear Fausto in Florence. He gave me a place to stay and came to find me when I got lost looking for the statue of David.

Luigi, my artist angel in Florence, walked with me around town so I wouldn't feel lonely.

In Rome, my angel Lorenzo invited me to be his guest at his restaurant. He made me feel comfortable with his delicious food and friendly company.

It was Gian Luca at the Hotel Igea in Rome who saved me a room and told me to be sure to throw 2 coins into Trevi Fountain so I would fall in love. He was also the angel that was so protective towards me.

I never had a single chance to feel lonely or uncomfortable or lost. Every one of these angels watched over me in Italy and gently guided me along my path to find Giovanni. I know I was given a miracle. If I hadn't been guided to Giovanni, I would not have known I had cancer. I would not have been able to catch it in time. I would not be a survivor.

There are people who don't believe in something unless it is scientifically proven. They will analyze this and come up with a logical explanation. Some may even think this was all a coincidence. Many people won't believe there are angels. But I know what I believe. You can't analyze miracles. You accept them and believe.

The Hebrew word for angel is mal'ak, which means to dispatch as a deputy; messenger; ambassador. The Greek word for angel is aggelos, which means to bring tidings, a messenger. The word angel is used, in one form or another, 198 times in the Bible.

"Let brotherly love continue. Be not forgetful to entertain strangers; for thereby some have entertained angels unawares." Hebrews 2,16

— CHAPTER FORTY-ONE —

Back To Rome

My husband and I recently took a vacation with another couple to England, France and Italy. No one knew it but this time when we were in Rome, I finally looked for Giovanni's face in the crowded city. I thought about what I would do if I found him.

I wanted to hug him and tell him how very sorry I was for hurting him years ago. I wanted him to know why I lied to him. I wanted him to tell me he was happy with someone else and tell him I was happy. I needed to tell him, "Thank you for saving my life." I suppose I needed to tell him, "Good Bye."

I walked up the Spanish Steps alone and looked out into the sea of faces below for his special face. "Where are you Giovanni?" kept playing over and over in my mind. I believed because it was something I wanted so badly that I would find him. He wasn't there. It began to rain. I opened my umbrella and slowly walked back down the steps. The gray skies matched my mood. I had expectations of finding him and talking with him here.

I looked at the faces of all the people I passed on the streets as I walked to Trevi Fountain. When I arrived, I sat there awhile and threw a coin in so I would return to Rome. I searched all the faces by the fountain. He loved this fountain. I really hoped he might be here. I couldn't find him.

When we went to Piazza Santa Maria in Trastevere, I went inside Santa Maria Church alone. There's a small box at the front of the church with a slot in it. Beside it are slips of paper to write someone's name on. They will say a prayer for this person. I wrote Giovanni Giovanetti on the small paper and put it in the slot. I sat on a wooden pew and prayed that Giovanni found love and happiness and was well. That's all I could do. I was 13 years too late. I never saw Giovanni again.

I remembered Evelyne asking me if I had called Giovanni at the end of my 11 months of treatments. At the time I felt I couldn't. I thought it was best for him to just let it be. Now I wish I had called him. He went through so much with me. I should have told him I survived.

I read somewhere that people come into our lives for a reason, a season or a lifetime. I know Giovanni came into my life on May 28, 1992 for a reason, for a season. I was the one, not him, who made the decision that he would not be with me for a lifetime because I believed my lifetime was ending.

I will never forgive myself for hurting Giovanni. I wish

I could somehow eliminate the pain from his life that I caused. I've been alive for the past 13 years because of him and he doesn't even know. Perhaps he'll read this book one day and forgive me. We all have to live with our choices and fortunately, I did live through mine.

— Chapter Forty-Two —

A Positive Future

For the past 13 years since I survived cancer, I have had so many fantastic and beautiful experiences. I have looked into the smiling eyes of the people in Thailand and enjoyed the tropical beauty of Singapore and Kuala Lumpur. I have talked with the friendly people in Vietnam. I met beautiful children in a small village in India who proudly wrote their names for me. I have seen a million stars over the desert in Oman and the ancient pyramids of Egypt.

I met a pretty young Bedouin woman in the incredibly beautiful lost city of Petra, Jordan. She liked my pink crystal earrings and I liked hers. They were handmade from small desert stones. We traded earrings. It's fun to think that she's wearing my earrings as she roams the desert.

In a tiny rustic village on the Amazon River I made friends with a small boy named Alex. I gave him fishing line and hooks for his dad. He took my hand and gave me a tour of his village. To thank him, I gave him a Mickey Mouse sucker and a quarter. The next day, when we returned to the village I saw him again. Someone had made a small hole in the quarter and put a string through it. Little 8-year old Alex was proudly wearing it as a necklace. Gerry called it his "Saint Susan" medal.

I had lunch in a 200 year old farmhouse with a family in Sweden. I rode a camel in Morocco and walked the entire wall surrounding Dubrovnik, Croatia. I have seen the sunrise in Machupicchu and wandered through ancient ruins in Turkey. I have met the friendliest people in the world in Australia and seen the snow, sparkling like diamonds in my own backyard.

The best things I have seen since my cancer recovery are the beautiful faces of my three grandchildren. Charissa, Matthew and Susie are my 3 little angels in Nevada.

I have seen such beauty and met so many good people from around the world. My dream was to see more of our world. My husband is making my dreams come true. All of these wonderful experiences were accomplishments in my life with him, after cancer. We still have many new adventures planned for a positive future together.

My battle with cancer and my love affair with a Roman are part of my past. That's all behind me now. I am living a new chapter in my life with Gerry. We just celebrated our 10-year wedding anniversary. We are having a terrific time on this adventure called life.

While struggling to write the story about my past, there were many times when I had to face my memories and I cried. I couldn't even write the words. I would have to walk away, sometimes for an hour, sometimes for days. Then that one question Evelyne asked me would start nagging me and wouldn't go away. "If it saved one person's life, would you do it?" and I knew I had to continue to the end. I asked God to help me with the words to make an impact on at least one woman so her life could be saved.

I don't know why I was chosen for the miracle I was given. I may never know. Perhaps a life will be saved because I wrote my story? I hope so.

I don't think of my story with Giovanni and wonder "What if?" or cry because it's over. I smile because it happened. I feel so fortunate to have been loved so much by him. Many people in their lifetime never get to experience the intensity of love that we felt for one another.

I will always cherish my memories of Giovanni and his Susanna.

The End